Multidisciplinary Working in Forensic Mental Health Care

Edited by

Stuart Wix CPNDip MA RMN RGN

Honorary Lecturer, University of Birmingham; Honorary Tutor, King's College London; Forensic Nurse Consultant, Reaside Clinic, Birmingham

Martin S. Humphreys BDS MB BS MRCPsych

Senior Lecturer in Forensic Psychiatry, University of Birmingham; Honorary Consultant Forensic Psychiatrist, Birmingham and Solihull Mental Health NHS Trust, Reaside Clinic, Birmingham

Foreword by

Herschel Prins MPhil Hon LL D

Professor, Midlands Centre for Criminology and Criminal Justice, University of Loughborough; Honorary Professor, School of Psychology, University of Birmingham

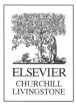

ELSEVIER
CHURCHILL
LIVINGSTONE

EDINBURGH   LONDON   NEW YORK   OXFORD   PHILADELPHIA   ST LOUIS   SYDNEY   TORONTO   2005

ELSEVIER
CHURCHILL
LIVINGSTONE

First published 2005

ISBN 0 443 07396 1

British Library Cataloguing in Publication Data
A catalogue record for this book is available from the British Library

Library of Congress Cataloging in Publication Data
A catalog record for this book is available from the Library of Congress

Notice
Knowledge and best practice in this field are constantly changing. As new research and experience broaden our knowledge, changes in practice, treatment and drug therapy may become necessary or appropriate. Readers are advised to check the most current information provided (i) on procedures featured or (ii) by the manufacturer of each product to be administered, to verify the recommended dose or formula, the method and duration of administration, and contraindications. It is the responsibility of the practitioner, relying on their own experience and knowledge of the patient, to make diagnoses, to determine dosages and the best treatment for each individual patient, and to take all appropriate safety precautions. To the fullest extent of the law, neither the publisher nor the editors assumes any liability for any injury and/or damage.

The Publisher

 ELSEVIER
your source for books,
journals and multimedia
in the health sciences
www.elsevierhealth.com

The
Publisher's
policy is to use
**paper manufactured
from sustainable forests**

Printed in China

Contents

Contributors

Jeff Baker BSc(Hons) CQSW
Senior Probation Officer, West Midlands Probation Service, Birmingham

Vincent Baxter BSc MSc RMN
Team Leader Community Forensic Nursing, Hatherton Centre, Stafford

Luke Birmingham MRCPsych MRCP MD
Senior Lecturer in Psychiatry, University of Southampton; Consultant Forensic Psychiatrist, Ravenswood House, Fareham, Hampshire

Gill Chalder MSc RMN (Forensic Mental Health)
Forensic Nurse Consultant, South Staffordshire Healthcare Trust, Stafford

Richard Gray DipHE BSc(Hons) MSCDLFHTM PhD RN
Lecturer and MRC Fellow in Health Service Research, Institute of Psychiatry, London

Nick Griffin MB ChB BSc FRC Psych
Consultant Forensic Psychiatrist, Director of Forensic Mental Health Services, South Staffordshire Healthcare Trust, Stafford

Rebecca A. Hills MSc DipCOT
Acute Services Manager, Millview Hospital, Hove, East Sussex

Aidan Houlders DMS MSc CQSW
Senior Social Worker, Reaside Clinic; Birmingham

Martin S. Humphreys BDS MB BS MRCPsych
Senior Lecturer in Forensic Psychiatry, University of Birmingham; Honorary Consultant Forensic

Psychiatrist, Reaside Clinic, Birmingham and Solihull Mental Health NHS Trust, Birmingham

Jason Jones BSc(Hons) ClinPsyD Cpsychol AFBPsS
Chartered Forensic and Clinical Psychologist, Reaside Clinic, Birmingham; Honorary Research Fellow, University of Birmingham, Birmingham

Jeremy Kenney-Herbert MB BS FRANZCP MRCPsych
Honorary Senior Lecturer, University of Birmingham; Consultant Forensic Psychiatrist, Reaside Clinic, Birmingham

Philip Kenny
Solicitor specialising in Mental Health Law, West Midlands

Kate Lyons DipManagement Studies BA(Hons)
Service Director, Men's Service, Broadmoor High Security Hospital, Crowthorne

Peter Nolan BA(Hons) BEd(Hons) MEd PhD RMN RGN DN RNT
South Staffordshire Mental Health Trust, Senior Lecturer, University of Stafford, Stafford

Carol Peckham BSc(Hons) RMN
Team Leader, Mental Health In-Reach Team, Her Majesty's Prison, Winchester

Chris Plowman BSc MSc ClinPsyD
Chartered Clinical Psychologist, Her Majesty's Prison, Birmingham

Sharon Riordan DipPsychology BA(Hons) MA
Lecturer in Forensic Mental Health Care, University of Birmingham, Birmingham

Deborah Robson DipHE BSc(Hons) RMN
*Tutor and Research Nurse in Medication
Management, Institute of Psychiatry, King's College,
London*

Stuart Wix CPNDip MA RMN RGN
*Honorary Lecturer, University of Birmingham;
Honorary Tutor, King's College London; Forensic
Nurse Consultant, Reaside Clinic, Birmingham and
Solihull NHS Mental Health Trust, Birmingham*

Foreword

The title of this multiauthored book encapsulates correctly the changes that have occurred in our thinking and activity within the field that used to be entitled forensic-psychiatry. This change in title reflects shifts in emphasis in a number of dimensions in the field. There is the increasing recognition that work with mentally disordered offenders needs to encompass a very wide range of disciplines if the many and varied needs of this group of individuals are to be met. Such an assortment of needs is very well described in the wide range of contributions assembled by the editors of this volume. The change of nomenclature also reflects the lessening of the primacy of medicine (in this case psychiatry) in this field. This trend in no way diminishes the importance of psychiatry, but serves to recognise the many-faceted elements in the challenges that offenders and offender-patients represent. And so, in this very useful collection of contributions we find a well-informed and catholic representation; for example, law, management, psychiatry, psychology, nursing, social work and probation, and pharmacy. Perhaps we are not yet sufficiently advanced to have a 'consumer' contribution, but no doubt such a contribution will find its place at some future date. The title chosen for the volume also reflects another trend, namely that of 'joined-up' government. The need for mutually supportive endeavour is apparent in the numerous central government memoranda issued in recent times. It is significant to note, for example, that the major conference called to launch the Government's proposals for managing individuals with dangerous severe personality disorder (DSPD) (a political *not* a clinical description) was attended by both the Secretary of State for Health and the Home Secretary. A further example of this trend is the very recent creation of the National Offender Management Service (NOMS). This brings together both prison and probation services in one correctional 'estate'. (The idea behind this development is, of course, not new; it was being mooted as long ago as the early 1960s during my own time in the Home Office Probation Inspectorate.) It should be noted that the various authors in this useful work make no extravagant claims for interdisciplinary working. They go as far as to state in all humility that there is 'limited evidence to demonstrate that team working improves the quality of care provided to the user of the service' (p. 20). This modest acknowledgement may well be true but the materials contained in this book certainly offer opportunities to improve upon the current 'state of the art'. In noting the complexities of the task so ably demonstrated in this volume perhaps we can be comforted by Alexander Pope's description of 'a mighty maze, but not without a plan.' (Essay on Man, Epistle 1 (1773) 1.1.).

Professor Herschel Prins
August, 2004

Preface

Forensic mental health services have been developing apace over the last decade or more and are principally concerned with the treatment and care of mentally disordered offenders and others who may require a similar form of approach. Treatment and care within the field are predominantly delivered in a collaborative, multidisciplinary way, and as such, are enhanced by the differing strengths of all of those who make up the multiprofessional team. Our purpose in producing this book has been to address some of the practical and theoretical issues which face all the disciplines involved in this form of working, be they practitioners who are new to the field or already well established. We would hope also to appeal to both undergraduate and postgraduate students undertaking studies in forensic mental health care, or mental health care in general, where many of the same principles apply, as well as those working in the many agencies linked with the criminal justice system who regularly come in to contact with mentally disordered offenders.

We have attempted to examine how effective multidisciplinary working can be achieved in clinical practice and proposed some systems and models of good practice to highlight this. The book places multidisciplinary working in forensic mental health care in an appropriate historical context. Our original motivation for seeking to write about multidisciplinary working in forensic mental health care arose as a result of what seemed to us to be the relative dearth of dedi-

cated texts available to clinicians working in this specific specialist area. We have actively sought to produce a text that addresses the subject matter covered from a range of different professional perspectives but not in an exclusive way.

The emphasis throughout the book has been to draw upon the expertise of as wide a group of contributors from around the United Kingdom as possible. This was our objective from the outset. We have included contributions, not only from a range of clinicians working in forensic settings, but also a number of non-clinical professionals, including a solicitor specialising in mental health law, a senior probation officer, an academic and a health service manager, whose unique involvement in the treatment and care of mentally disordered offenders, in its broadest sense, hopefully will provide the reader with a more complete picture of the potential for multidisciplinary working in action. Additionally, it has been our aim to integrate some original research findings pertinent to the subject, as well as case study examples, to provide a sense of perspective to the reader.

There are sections within the book that we hope might also have some international appeal, particularly those chapters which cover theoretical foundations, issues to do with risk assessment, the important business of team building as well as treatment planning and the relatively new concept of medication management. These not only provide an overview of their respective subject areas, but also illustrate practical examples and applications in day-to-day clinical practice. We have aimed to create a book that is also 'user friendly', one that is not overly academic in style but equally not too simplistic. Lastly we would like to think that what we have produced here is a starting point, rather than an end in itself, for those involved in the field and that it might act as a catalyst to others, not simply as a means of improving clinical practice but also to further exploration, research and writing about truly integrated multidisciplinary working in forensic mental health care.

Stuart Wix
Martin S. Humphreys
Birmingham 2004

Acknowledgements

We would like to thank Julie Evans, Kerrie Hughes and Tracey Hayes for their considerable and combined efforts in preparing the many drafts for this book. We would also like to extend our thanks to the contributors who are all experienced in the field, and for their willingness in applying themselves to the task of writing about their work. We are also extremely grateful to every one at Elsevier.

Chapter 1

The historical context

Peter Nolan

INTRODUCTION

Although academics on both sides of the Atlantic have discussed the history of the public asylums from a variety of perspectives, the social function of the criminal lunatic asylum has been little investigated. Prior (1997) considers the forensic mental health care services to have been sadly neglected by historians, a neglect which has contributed to the public's lack of sympathy with them and those who use it. However, we do know something of both the 18th century subscription asylums and the 19th century county lunatic asylums, about the types of patients admitted there, the treatments provided and the ways in which different institutions were managed (Porter, 1987; 1995). Even though general mental health and forensic services are today in many ways clearly distinguished, this was not always the case. There was a time when they were synonymous, and criminal lunatics and those suffering with mild mental health problems, such as depression, were housed together in the same facilities or on the same wards as those who had been before the courts. In 1837, the Hereford Lunatic Asylum was condemned by magistrates for its inadequate facilities for *criminal and non-criminal lunatics* (Smith, 1999). Allegations of mismanagement and neglect included reference to poorly trained staff, the lack of active therapeutic regimes, overuse of restraints and punishments, such as cold baths, and poor record keeping. The Asylum was threatened with non-renewal of its licence unless it improved its facilities and procedures. Long after forensic services were separated from general mental health services, problems have continued to be identified in both sectors; in the forensic field as witnessed by the inquiries into the Special Hospitals at Broadmoor, Ashworth and Rampton over a century and a half later (Parker, 1985; Snowden and Freeman, 1999). This chapter presents a broad picture of the history of forensic mental health care, using available evidence to examine how various types of collaboration and multidisciplinary working have shaped the focus of care available in the field today. The reader should be cautioned at the outset against the ever-present danger of imposing on the past our own current values and meanings. Dingwall et al. (1988) alert us to the *nominal fallacy* of applying modern concepts and ideas expressed in today's systems and structures to the past, and proceeding as if terms have been used consistently throughout history. This is most definitely not so in health care, in general, and perhaps even less so in forensic mental health care, in particular.

Of all the services available within the NHS, forensic mental health care is arguably the most contested and least understood, even among health professionals. It is a minority service within a service and has long suffered from underfunding, public stigma and isolation from other parts of the health care system. Forensic services care for some of the most marginalised, vulnerable and difficult to treat individuals in society. Many patients may be inaccurately described as demonstrating negative behaviours, such as violence, duplicity and unpredictability, while having self-care patterns that clearly compromise their ability to make independent choices in their lives (Campbell et al., 2000). While periods of inpatient care now tend to consist of only a brief episode in hospital, of weeks rather than months for the vast majority of mental health patients, those admitted to forensic facilities may spend an average of 18 months or more as inpatients and, in some cases, in excess of 3 years. During this episode, patients are confined, closely observed by staff, and have little or no control over who they associate with. The needs of female patients and those from ethnic minorities have been found to be even more poorly met in forensic services than in mental health care in general. Although the range and type of treatments offered are important, as with other mental health service users, it is the quality of relationships formed with staff that is the strongest determinant of successful outcome (Nolan et al., 1999). Unfortunately, in forensic settings, staff who have ideally been recruited for their therapeutic skills may spend much of their time gathering data required by the courts or other outside agencies. Indeed, in many instances, attending to legal and related matters is what differentiates the work of forensic personnel from that of other mental health workers.

THE NATURE AND DEFINITION OF FORENSIC MENTAL HEALTH CARE

Although various forms of forensic care exist worldwide, they are more strongly established in Europe and in countries that have adopted European systems of justice and health service provision (Skultans, 1979; Snowden and Freeman, 1999). Forensic mental health care has emerged from an alliance—some would argue an uneasy one—between psychiatry and the legal system. On the one hand, it is multidisciplinary and has always been so, yet it remains a separate subsystem within health care. It is understandable that the public and some health professionals find it difficult to distinguish between general and forensic mental health services when nearly half the patients currently on acute admission wards in some parts of the United Kingdom are detained under a section of the Mental Health Act (Bowers et al., 1999). Recently, policy initiatives, instigated by the Home Office and the Department of Health, have tried to ensure that developments in the one service influence what happens in the other.

History suggests that, whereas legislation can be enacted and institutions built, almost overnight, it takes time and effort to establish a branch of health care that commands the respect of the public as well as meeting the needs of individuals. The threat to society posed by the refractory behaviour of certain people has long been recognised, but it was not until the 18th century that separate facilities began to emerge for those whose bad behaviour might be attributed to madness (Skultans, 1979; Porter, 1995). The mere provision of institutions created the opportunity to build a specialist branch of health care but, more importantly, people with vision and compassion were required, people who were able to identify the effective components of the care provided. It has taken years of careful observation and intelligent analysis to reach our present understanding, however limited that still might be, of the multiple and complex problems faced by mentally disordered offenders. Services originally located in institutions characterised as 'benign warehouses', built to appease public anxiety, and where care was primarily defined as containment and treatment as pharmacological intervention, have now given way to integrated services that seek to address the psychological, physical, social and spiritual needs of people (Mercer et al., 2000). The contribution of individual disciplines to forensic mental health care has been considerable, but working together, they have been found to have a far more powerful impact on patients.

This is not to say that the historical tension in forensic services between care and containment no longer exists (Porter, 2002). Commentators continue to refer to the difficulty in finding the balance between the two. Some have been of the opinion that a legal straight-jacket thwarts the creation of a therapeutic infrastructure in forensic services (Unsworth, 1987); yet Bean (1985) has argued that psychiatrists and others working in the field require some form of external surveillance to ensure that they do not exceed their legal powers. Forensic mental health care may be seen as a medicolegal approach to identifying and meeting people's needs; psychiatrists aim to elicit a diagnosis while the law seeks to establish the extent to which persons can be held responsible for their actions. This collaboration has become established over the years as both medicine and the law have attempted to respond to human catastrophes involving mentally disordered offenders. Unsworth (1987) noted, however, that the supposed equality between the disciplines of law and psychiatry has not always been manifest. During the latter part of the 19th, and for most of the 20th century, for instance, psychiatrists have tended to leave most of the decision-making to lawyers and have been reluctant to be drawn into conflict with them. In 1976, in the case of Peter Sutcliffe, known as the 'Yorkshire Ripper', all of the doctors who examined agreed that he was psychotic, with clear delusional beliefs. In court, however, they were made to look foolish under cross-examination and Sutcliffe was sent to prison (Snowden and Freeman, 1999). After further psychiatric assessment, once the public horror surrounding the case had subsided, Sutcliffe was in fact confirmed to be suffering from schizophrenia and transferred to a special hospital.

Forensic mental health care professionals have become engaged in an ongoing debate to establish what is meant by reasonable or unreasonable behaviour, with the definition changing in accordance with the values prevailing in society at any given time. Equally problematic is setting up legal processes to judge whether certain behaviours are reasonable or not. Critics argue that no matter how robust and transparent the system of justice, it can never be value free. There is always scope for doubt and error. In reviewing the history of rationalism, Porter (2002) asks 'What is reason?', 'What is madness?' and 'Where lie the dividing lines?' He offers an amusing anecdote which concerns the Restoration playwright, Nathaniel Lee, who on being brought into custody, complained, 'They called me mad. I called them mad and damn them, they outvoted me!' Philosophers such as Erasmus and Robert Burton considered that human beings have to learn the benefits of reason by first experiencing the chaos of devoting their lives to satisfying their passions. They contended that civilisation itself, far from being a stronghold against unreason and emotional instability, is their precipitant. On that basis, one might argue that, in treating mental disorder, a certain section of society punishes with psychotherapeutics vulnerable souls that it has previously driven to distraction.

The concept of 'forensic care' can evoke strong negative feelings in people who are normally rational, objective and fair-minded. Studies have reported that staff can be every bit as repulsed by patients and their behaviour as the general public (Thomsen et al., 1999). In common with other low-status branches of health care, forensic services have long suffered from public disinterest other than at times of catastrophe, lack of strong leadership, inadequate funding and most significantly, from being stigmatised by other health care professionals as having more in common with the penal than the health care system. Public inquiries into the running of forensic services often reinforce public antipathy towards forensic patients and those who care for them. Such antipathy has even today, to be combated when endeavouring to improve conditions and services for mentally disordered offenders. The tendency to emphasise public safety at the expense of individual rights is as prevalent today as it was in the past (Morrison, 1990).

Attempting to define the province of forensic mental health care remains problematic. Recent policy statements are far from unanimous in their definitions. Mason (2002) has demonstrated that the term 'forensic care' is used differently by different groups and agencies, and is indeed one that not all interested parties accept as useful or worth retaining. Taborda and Abdalla-Filho (2002) contend that the service comprises all aspects of care that are in direct service to the courts either before or after sentencing. Extending this definition, Lonsdale (2001) states that the service includes those who work with victims and witnesses, as well as those involved with suspects and known perpetrators of violence, including sexual assault, and others who assist with the investigation of deaths and the work of coroners. Woods (2002) adopts a definition of forensic care that includes creating a safe and therapeutic environment, encompasses risk and anger management, and which uses offence-focused interventions and avoids labelling.

Mason (2002) finds that forensic care is rooted in the medicalisation of criminology that proposes that there is a relationship between mental disorder and offending behaviour. Knowles (2003) argues that the term 'psychopathic disorder', as used in the 1959 and 1983 Mental Health Acts, is contentious and is a legal term rather than a clinical diagnosis. Gove and Georges (2001) remark that forensic care can only be defined within the context of the laws that govern a country. Although many countries have similar principles underpinning their statutory and case law, their practical approaches to care and custody can be completely different. In some countries, forensic services are involved in legal executions (Halpern and Freedman, 2002), evaluating the sequelae of torture (Wenzel, 2002), and monitoring and assessing the effects of terrorism and bioterrorism (Baum and Dougal, 2002).

Nursing authors tend to refer to the definition of the International Association of Forensic Nurses (1999), which states:

> The forensic nurse provides direct services to individual clients, consultation services to nursing, medical, and law related agencies, as well as providing expert testimony in areas dealing with questioned death, adequacy of service delivery and specialised diagnoses of specific conditions related to nursing.

This clearly defines the provision of forensic services first and foremost in relation to the legal system, although other authorities would argue that nursing encompasses all that is provided therapeutically to those in receipt of forensic care (Mercer et al., 2000). There does, despite these apparent differences, seem to be general agreement that the service is triangular in nature, involving relationships between the carer, the patient, and either the judiciary or the prison system.

Further study is required of those who have been labelled 'mad' *and* 'bad', and of the social attitudes to crime and mental illness that have prevailed at different periods. Examining the history of forensic services should lead to a better understanding of their evolution and of the origins of contemporary tensions that lie at the heart of forensic mental health care.

IN SEARCH OF THE ROOTS OF FORENSIC CARE

Historians have tended to open their accounts of the development of mental health care, in accordance with their individual ideas of the significant. Many are eager to discuss the views of both Greeks and Romans on practices around the management of the mentally disordered. The Ancients endeavoured to prevent the insane person from destroying life, limb and property, and attributed total responsibility for them to their families or guardians (Berrios, 1996; Porter, 2002). 'If a man is mad', stated Plato in *The Laws*, 'he shall not be at large in the city, but his family shall keep him in any way they can.' Insanity remained a domestic responsibility for many centuries and, in some parts of the world, most notably in Japan, until well into the 20th century. Those deemed to be a high risk to others were confined at home, whilst those less afflicted were permitted to go out only if accompanied. The mad were shunned because of the belief that they were possessed by evil spirits, which could fly out of them and take hold over others (Porter, 2002). Christ sent the evil spirits that had possessed the man whose relatives sought His help into a herd of swine and drove the swine over a cliff.

Roman attitudes towards the mentally disordered were generally less punitive than those of the Greeks. They cherished a romantic belief that those 'whom the gods favour, they make mad'. Under Roman law in early England, the insane offender was treated with leniency, on the basis that the madness from which he suffered was in itself sufficient punishment. This position seems to have held for several hundred years. In the 13th century, it was stated that the 'will to harm' must be present for an offence to have been committed and that without such 'will', the accused could not be held responsible. Skultans (1979) shows how the definition of a sane or reasonable person that prevailed in Europe for many centuries incorporated notions of discipline and self-control. The sane man kept his reason, emotions, judgement and discernment under the control of his will. Insane persons, by contrast, were victims of their passions and were powerless to do anything about them. They shared much in common with animals, namely an inability to learn from experience, unpredictability and a propensity to indulge in aggressive outbursts. Not only were their lives miserable but so were the lives of their families and those around them.

We know that, in Britain, from about the 6th to the 16th centuries, peripatetic monks helped with the management of the 'spiritually bewildered' and those who suffered from accidie—the belief that life was not worth living (Clarke, 1975). Where individuals were distraught or could not be restrained from harm, they were removed to the monasteries where they were encouraged to live the 'ordered' life of the monks until they had regained order in their own lives. The first legislation allowing the confinement of people deemed to be dangerous was enacted in 1482. Such individuals could be incarcerated, in the interests of public safety, either in their own homes or in local Bridewells (Alderidge, 1979). No reference was made to how their time while thus confined should be spent nor under what circumstances they might be released.

The Vagrancy Act of 1744 required that those who were 'furiously mad and dangerous' should be detained for the public good. They might be incarcerated either in prisons or in asylums. Both kinds of institutions might also house debtors, minor felons and the mildly mentally ill as well as the criminally insane (Smith, 1999; Unsworth, 1987). They were poorly managed, squalid and inhumane. In Worcester, the prison was one of the sights of the City. On Assizes Sunday, the Sunday during or immediately following the Assizes prisoners were shown to the crowds. Visitors would give 6d to the gaoler to point out to them those condemned to be executed (Porter, 1987). Inside the prison, debtors and felons were separated only by an ironwork grille and could communicate freely. Visitors to felons were searched but not those to debtors. The debtors' common room was tiny and was also used as a chapel. There was no special room for the condemned criminal; by day, he was chained to a post near to the door of the common room/chapel. There was a regular transfer of prisoners to the 'transports' in Bristol, from where they were shipped to the plantations. In 1783, the prison suffered an outbreak of gaol fever following which the County magistrates spent £3431 on its improvement. However, the building was old and insecure, and there were numerous escapes over the next 20 years. Proposals to build a new establishment were put forward in 1802, but the landowners from both the county and the city protested at the expense involved and the plans were shelved. In 1807, Chief Baron MacDonald arrived at Worcester for the Assizes and found that the prisoners who were the accused in the most important cases had vanished. His Lordship warned the Grand Jury that the County would be heavily fined if matters were not put right. A new prison was at last built and opened in Salt Lane in 1813 (Smith, 1999).

Appalling conditions in the prisons finally led to action on the part of the public-spirited. John Howard, born in 1726 and appointed sheriff of Bedfordshire in 1773, was the most eminent of the reformers. It is after him that the Howard League for Penal Reform is named. A man of great piety and founder of the Howard Congregational Church in Mill Street in Bedford, Howard believed that his Christian beliefs demanded social commitment. He was particularly concerned with the incidence of gaol fever (typhus) and madness in the prisons and felt that more than medicine was needed to address these evils. Typhus was frequently referred to as the 'prisoners' friend' as it shortened lives and hence the time they had to endure prison conditions (Smith, 1981). Howard recognised that madness was induced or exacerbated by the trauma of incarceration and fear. He campaigned to reduce overcrowding, to improve prisoners' hygiene and diet, and to secure for them more fresh air and exercise.

Howard was not the only humanitarian in the field. Thomas Arnold, Superintendent at the subscription asylum in Leicester, aimed to find a balance between security and compassion, although he still believed that it was important to subdue and control the recalcitrant before they could benefit from being in an institution. Once they had been made to submit, kindness and reform might follow (Carpenter, 1989). During the latter part of the 18th century, Arnold was regarded as one of the foremost thinkers on the management of criminal lunatics in England. He vigorously combated what he saw as interference from laymen, especially local magistrates, who until 1889 were the real managers of public asylums. Like other Superintendents, he resented the surveillance role of magistrates and their ability to over-rule his authority. By the mid-1790s, Arnold had lost interest in this work, perhaps disillusioned that so few inmates improved or recovered, and the Leicester asylum deteriorated (Smith, 1999).

The brainchild of Jeremy Bentham (1748–1832) was the *panopticon*, an institution built to maximise observation of those within it. Bentham believed that recalcitrants needed to be subjected to a totalitarian regime until they were able to manage themselves. He viewed asylums as models for a moral utopia. It was his opinion that the role of asylum doctors was to abolish barbarous practices and analyse madness in order to cure it. Placing madmen in the ordered rational world of the asylum was the precondition, which would facilitate the cure (Scull, 1977). Bentham devised rules for asylum management and living:

- *The Rule of Leniency*: no person in the institution should have to endure gratuitous suffering, and managers had a duty to prevent abuse and neglect and address them whenever they were found.
- *The Rule of Severity* (or the rule of less eligibility): the care provided for inmates should be no more than an ordinary poor person would receive outside the institution.
- *The Rule of Economy*: as the main purpose of the institution was punishment, it should be run as cheaply as possible.

Bentham's thinking typified the ongoing tension in these institutions between compassion and punishment. Despite expressing and demonstrating considerable humanity, he nonetheless advocated that feeding of inmates should be kept to a minimum so as not to encourage malingering. He was also a firm supporter of 'hard labour' and 'walking the treadmill'.

In 1859, Thomas Guy, for whom Guy's Hospital in London is named, was appointed medical Superintendent to Milbank Prison. He soon became critical of previous influences in prisons. He combated the widely held belief that those kept in secure environments were inferior in mind and body to the rest of the population and, therefore, had less need for nutrition, education and comfort. His observations led him to conclude that secure institutions were beyond reform while they remained isolated, self-perpetuating and insular systems (Porter, 1995). In 1803 he wrote:

> Nothing is worse than suffering from a nervous imagination and mental turmoil, and there are many people here who suffer from both; there are no cures.

In his opinion, the purpose of asylums and prisons was to re-Christianise the fallen. He recognised that nothing was being done to address the mental state of prisoners and asylum inmates, even if their physical needs were being met.

Elizabeth Fry campaigned on behalf of women prisoners. A regular visitor to Newgate, she recommended that female prison officers should oversee inmates and that female visitors in turn should oversee them. Her interest was borne out of personal experience of mental illness, notably depression, for which she was confined on 11 occasions during the course of her life (Black, 1990).

At the beginning of the 19th century, debate was rife regarding separate establishments for criminal lunatics. Following the County Asylums Act of 1808 which authorised the detention of all insane people to new institutions, the governors of the Bethlem Hospital entered into negotiation with the Corporation of London regarding a new hospital to be built in St Georges's Fields, Southwark. On the 25th August 1810, the Home Office wrote to the governors to enquire whether they would set aside part of the new site for a criminal lunatic asylum. The governors were assured that the erection of buildings and the maintenance of the inmates, including their funeral expenses, would be paid for out of public funds. The governors agreed, only stipulating that the new department should be under their absolute control and not subject to visits from county magistrates. Two buildings, one accommodating 45 males and the other 15 females, were completed and occupied on 31st October 1816 (O'Donoghue, 1914). By 1844, there were 85 criminal patients there while, elsewhere in England; there was provision for 224 such cases in various asylums. Although it was now increasingly recognised that there was a need to cater separately for the criminally insane and that the accommodation at the Bethlem was inadequate, it was not until 1848 that another special ward was built at Fisherton House near Salisbury.

Dr Francis White argued vigorously in favour of making special provision for criminal lunatics. He was the first Inspector for Lunatics in Ireland and, from this position of authority, put forward his arguments to the Lord Chancellor for separate services. These included the fact that there was insufficient accommodation for pauper lunatics in Ireland at the time, that it would be cost effective to have all criminal lunatics in one place, guaranteeing the public greater safety, and that outsiders could be prohibited from visiting for reasons of morbid curiosity. White also suggested that having special facilities on both sides of the water would enable Irish criminal lunatics to be sent to England and vice versa, thus providing even better security! (Prior, 1997).

The strongest impetus for the provision of separate secure facilities came following the murder of the Prime Minister's Private Secretary by Daniel McNaughten in 1843. McNaughten was found not guilty on the grounds of insanity. His case gave rise to the legal rules in such circumstances still in use today (Carpenter, 1997). Another landmark case was that of Alexander Dingwall, who in Scotland in 1851 murdered his wife under the influence of drink. He had a long history of alcoholism. In his summing up, the judge referred to 'extenuating circumstances'. Over time, this precedent led to the development of the defence of 'diminished responsibility' and was eventually adopted in England in 1957 (Snowden and Freeman, 1999).

These and other such cases highlighted the need for suitable hospital provision for those who became embroiled in the criminal justice process but who were mentally unwell. As a result, Broadmoor Special Hospital was opened in 1863 in Berkshire, Rampton in Nottinghamshire in 1912 and Moss Side near Liverpool in 1919 to provide (high-security) hospital care to patients. They were managed and funded directly by central government. In the 20th century, nurses who worked in the special hospitals tended to belong to the Prison Officers' Association and to identify strongly with security services rather than with nursing. The special hospitals focused on security and surveillance rather then treatment. In

1981, so poor had conditions become at Rampton that the licence to train nurses was withdrawn, thus plunging the hospital into a staffing crisis that took some years to overcome (Hamilton, 1985). Male patients outnumbered females and records show that, at least in their early years, the inmates of the special hospitals were poorly educated, poverty-stricken and had little or no prospect of work (Prior, 1997). However, at least some of the staff that managed the patients on a day-to-day basis believed that rehabilitation was possible. Nevertheless medical explanations of deviant behaviour were sometimes ignored in favour of social ones. Good behaviour on the part of patients and manifestations of remorse for what they had done led to early discharge.

THE START OF FORENSIC SERVICES IN THE UK

In 1841, the Medico-Psychological Association (MPA) was founded at the instigation of Dr Hitch, resident Superintendent at the Gloucester Asylum, where the first meeting of this new organisation was held. In 1853, the Association began to publish the *Asylum Journal,* soon to be renamed the *Journal of Mental Science.* Doctors were invited to submit scholarly papers, which would help in building up the new discipline of 'psychiatry', a term first used in 1846. Of particular interest were papers describing psychiatric conditions and problems concerned with the running of large institutions. Heated debates regularly took place between competing schools of thought. At the forefront of such debate were psychiatrists from the universities of Glasgow and Edinburgh. Edinburgh University's first Professor of Medical Jurisprudence, Andrew Duncan, published widely, keenly aware that doctors were poorly prepared to give psychiatric evidence in the courts. In Duncan's experience, lawyers were far more influential than doctors in determining the outcome of cases relating to criminal lunatics. Duncan's colleague, John Pagan, wrote *Medical Jurisprudence,* one of the first textbooks on forensic medicine, based on a series of lectures he had delivered since the early 1830s. The book is still an eloquent argument for expert medical testimony to be accorded equal status with legal evidence (Andrews, 1997).

At Glasgow Royal Hospital, Yellowlees and his successors were also extending the debate about criminal lunacy. He believed that all mental illness was attributable to brain injury, and that careful examination of patients and recording of observations were the most important aspects of a doctor's role. He condemned the slack attitude towards notetaking that prevailed in some Scottish hospitals and argued that psychiatry would never become a respectable discipline if rigorous standards for the examination of patients were not enforced. Among the many physicians who came under his influence were the Edinburgh doctors, Skae and Laycock, who frequently published in the *Journal of Mental Science* in favour of greater reliance on expert medical testimony in the courts (Robinson, 1988).

Sir David Henderson formulated the concept of 'psychopathy' in the first half of the 20th century, again in Edinburgh. He spoke of how the individual is shaped by both heredity and the environment, and opposed the idea that certain characters could only deteriorate with no hope of rehabilitation. The term *psychopathic disorder* is still used today, but according to Snowden and Freeman (1999), in at least three different ways; as a legal classification in terms of the 1983 Mental Health Act; a clinical diagnosis, and a pejorative label. The term is often employed simply to identify truculent or difficult individuals, many of whom appear to be resistant to treatment.

During the 1930s, the age-old debate around the issue of free will and determinism was raised again in the context of the provision of mental health services. Those who upheld the notion that all individuals were free to make choices and, therefore, could and should be held accountable for their actions, saw prison as the most obvious holding place for mentally ill offenders. Foremost among this group was Dr Peter Scott. However, Scott felt that, although offenders deserved punishment, many could also benefit from treatment. He recommended setting up treatment units in prisons, which could help relieve the chronic overcrowding in the special hospitals. Despite his eloquence, Scott was unable to convince his colleagues of the validity of his idea. It was not until 1962 that Grendon Underwood Prison started to provide treatment for some prisoners along psychotherapeutic lines, followed a little later by Barlinnie Prison in Glasgow.

Like Scott, the psychiatrist, Hamblin Smith, also argued that punishment alone was not an adequate response to crime and might be inappropriate in the case of mentally ill offenders. He favoured separate forensic units in prisons where people would be seen as patients rather than prisoners and treatment rather than punishment would be the primary goal. Smith was supported by Hubert, a psychiatrist at St Thomas' Hospital, London, who argued from his experience of treating forensic patients that a psychotherapeutic approach resulted in a favourable outcome for many. The work of Smith and Hubert came to the attention of the Ministry of Health of the time. The government subsequently sanctioned the setting up of the *Institute for the Study and Treatment of Delinquency* (ISTD) in London in the late 1930s by Edward Glover. Glover promoted the view that there was a therapeutic alternative to prison and that a humane approach to the care of mentally ill offenders, coupled with education to increase self-awareness, would enable people to be reformed (Snowden and Freeman, 1999).

New ideas about what to do with mentally ill offenders influenced those charged with drawing up new mental health law. The 1959 Mental Health Act was hailed as an innovative piece of legislation that explicitly affirmed that mentally ill patients could be treated successfully and restored to their normal lives. This turned around the 1890 Lunacy Act that had considered magistrates best placed to make decisions about the mentally ill and which had presumed that few would recover sufficiently to be able to resume their previous lives. The 1959 Act was revolutionary in devising the category of 'voluntary patient' to describe those who themselves sought help for their illnesses and were willing to enter hospital of their own free will rather than being detained under the Act.

While the Act made access to care much easier and less stigmatising for many mentally ill people, facilities and treatment for mentally disordered offenders remained appallingly inadequate by contrast. The Butler Report of 1975 highlighted the 'yawning gap' in forensic mental health care services and recommended the development of medium secure units that would be the focus for the development of specialist practice (Bluglass, 1985). It urged that there should be more academic interest in the field and that a programme of research should be developed along with clinical provision. The first Professor of Forensic Psychiatry was Dr Gibbens, appointed to the Maudsley Hospital in 1975. As early as 1951, he had advocated for court-based mental health services, but it was not until 40 years later that mentally disordered offenders were diverted from the criminal justice system to the health services (Snowden and Freeman, 1999). The developments of links with academic institutions created the conditions in which research and multidisciplinary collaboration could be fostered. The creation of 'interim' and 'medium secure units' provided material for research and the inclusion of psychologists in the forensic care team boosted the amount of academic investigation being undertaken in secure environments. Nurses, occupational therapists and social workers also became involved in research, which sought to understand patients and their problems, and thereby improve the efficiency and efficacy of services.

Berrios (1996) has more recently suggested that more historical research is needed to explore how terms once used in psychiatry relate to those in use today. He questions whether the old notion of *moral insanity* has been subsumed into the more recent one of *psychopathic behaviour* and whether the words currently in favour are any better than those previously in vogue, such as *moral insanity, impulsion, impulsive insanity, lucid insanity* and *reasoning insanity*. Dingwall et al. (1988) have questioned whether we are talking about the same pathology and now, as before, even as terminology changes, whether in fact the pathology itself is different. Fashionable new intellectual ideas rather than empirical research may determine approaches to the criminally mentally ill. Thus, after the concept of free will fell out of fashion, volitional models of psychopathy disappeared. Likewise, new developments in psychiatry were fuelled by the work of Freud. Current explanations of deviant behaviour are a return to earlier views according to which both normal and abnormal behaviour may be dependent upon specific neurobiological events. Commentators point to the fact that what passes for 'assessment' of patients or 'diagnosis' are in essence an attempt to define what forensic care means at any point in history (Bowden, 1991).

HISTORY AND ITS IMPLICATIONS FOR MODERN FORENSIC CARE

As can be seen from this brief account, the history of forensic care is in part a history of definitions and in part a history of the management of the criminally insane. The care of such people has been, and remains, a mixture of the legal and clinical, as well as political. At any point in time, the government of the day, the efforts of those who have advocated on behalf of patients, and public opinion have determined forensic mental health policy. As with other branches of health care, it is also the history of how and why treatments were devised, the degree to which they were implemented and their eventual decline in order to give way to other forms of treatment. Differences of opinion regarding the treatment of mentally ill offenders have always existed between institutions, between doctors, between Boards of Governors and, above all, between magistrates and the law. During the 19th century, it was the courts that determined the running of the institutions even though it was the Medical Superintendents who had overall responsibility for standards of care and treatment.

Unsworth's (1987) historical review of services concludes that forensic institutions have always been unsure about their purpose, although security and containment remain a priority. Should they, he asks, have responsibility for testing new forms of treatment? Should they be engaged in research and education? And should they seek more integration with other forms of health care? The early special hospitals were isolated both geographically, to some extent, socially and professionally and their values and practices went unchallenged. Modern forensic units are smaller, and are encouraged to adopt approaches to their work that are similar to those in use by health care personnel elsewhere. Corrigan and McCracken (1995), however, have found that some units are just as detached from mainstream services as were the older ones; a *minority mentality* exists where individuals look to each other for support and leadership, rather than outside and beyond their own immediate environment. Lack of access to policymakers renders both patients and staff powerless in moulding the system to their needs. When units feel they are being scrutinised, they may tend to interact only within their own peer group and isolate themselves from the others (Hogg and Vaughan, 1995). Despite the many inquiries and directives, and the adoption of therapeutic language, forensic units still appear to find it difficult to embrace progressive practices. Tajfel and Turner (1979) have suggested that this is because the objectives of forensic care are unclear and that it is, therefore, very difficult to bring about change when people do not share the same view of their work. Sedgwick (1982) also considered that repeated attempts to change the culture of forensic care have failed because it incorporates multiple cultures rather than a single one. The various groups who work in the field of forensic mental health—psychiatrists, psychologists, social workers, nurses and occupational therapists—have each defined their own approach in contrast to, rather than in collaboration with, that of others. There is, therefore, the constant danger that some will see their contribution as more important than that of others (Conacher, 1993). As a consequence, they may see patients at the time of *their* choosing, see them independently, keep separate notes and fail to take account of other forms of treatment. This attitude may also extend to the notion that some questions and issues are more important than others, and equally some forms of research are more worthwhile and valid than others.

Nettleton (1995) states that health care has always been a stage where professionals jostle for power, prestige, status and recognition. It could be argued that competition is a controlling device and that tension is healthy for the survival of an organisation. However, competition may result in resources and energy being squandered on self-promotion to the detriment of patient care. In forensic settings, the dominance of the biomedical model is sustained through its close alliance with the law, while psychology has sought to assert itself through the alliance with research and education. Beyond the immediate context in which services are provided are international forces, which act mainly to reinforce medical dominance (Turner, 1987). A highly influential and powerful 'psychiatric-industrial complex', with a globalising base in the USA, not only seeks to expand its remit in relation to serious mental illness, but also to promote the psychiatrisation of 'minor' distress through branded drugs such as Prozac, Viagra and Ritalin.

Considering mental health services in this wider context, Carpenter (2000) notes that fiscal pressures started to bite following the oil crisis years of the mid-1970s and have certainly precipitated the rationalisation of mental health care. A medically dominated, 'downsized' psychiatric system has given increasing priority to containment of seriously disordered people, partly driven by public concerns about risk and 'dangerousness'. Carpenter describes how the adoption of therapeutic language and the 'softer' features of psychiatric intervention detract attention from forensic practice, even in a postasylum setting. The emphasis on containment and punishment over welfare, coupled with a declining or even 'zero tolerance' of all forms of deviance, are features of neoliberalism worldwide. The capacity of forensic mental health services to deliver restorative treatment is questioned by sceptics when most discharged patients progress to further supervised care in the community rather then re-entering the labour market.

Stone (1994) claims that the most significant problem facing providers of contemporary forensic services is the lack of ethical guidelines for how they should relate to patients and particularly for what they should say in the courtroom. Appelbaum (1997) argues that health professionals should stay out of the courtroom, as this is not an appropriate arena for them. Both these authors state that truth telling and respect for persons are the key principles upon which forensic services should be built. Gunn (2000) contends that, while different professionals may work to different values, the code of medical ethics should prevail in the forensic care team because it is the psychiatrist who takes responsibility for selecting a course of treatment and who usually appears in court. This argument may be at the heart of why multidisciplinary teamwork can be compromised in today's forensic services. Team meetings and discussions cannot mask the lack of genuine parity among the groups involved. Consultants in Forensic Psychiatry (of whom there were only eight at the time of the Butler Report in 1975, but who now number 150) in their statutory role of Responsible Medical Officer, and social workers as social supervisors, for instance, but nurses and occupational therapists have less statutory responsibility and may be excluded from decision-making (Coffey and Jenkins, 2002). The dominance of the biomedical model represented by the consultant psychiatrist remains a central plank upon which services are built and this situation inevitably presents an obstacle to more integrative working with other agencies (Stone, 1997).

CONCLUSIONS

So far, this chapter has focused on health professionals and systems of care with little or no reference to the user's viewpoint. Forensic services patients or clients have rarely been consulted about their perceptions of their own best interests. For this reason, Peter Thompson's book *Bound for Broadmoor* (1972) is especially valuable. Here he describes in detail what it was like to be in Broadmoor Hospital: the oppressive environment, the rigid routines, the pervading sense of hopelessness, and the long periods when there was no one to speak to. He explains why it is difficult to engage public interest in the plight of the criminally ill:

> The ordinary person, no matter how sympathetic or liberal, cannot be expected to visualise the circumstances of a mentally ill offender. People find it hard to think of inmates as people, or their disorders as very often caused, or at least aggravated, by contemporary public and social attitudes towards the mentally ill.
>
> (Thompson, 1972)

Thompson describes how he saw little evidence of staff collaboration, largely owing to the universal deference towards doctors. He regularly had interactions with doctors, psychologists, social workers and nurses, but it was evident that none of them consulted with each other because each frequently requested the same information. It was in spite of the system, rather than because of it, that some members of staff demonstrated kindness and sensitivity. He recalls very clearly the one doctor, and the nurses, who took time to be with him during periods of depression and loneliness. Mercer et al. (2000) state that the introduction of psychodynamic and behavioural therapies in the early 1970s in English special hospitals was instrumental in assisting staff to see the importance of interpersonal relationships with patients. As Sacks (1983) describes, such contact is invaluable:

> If we wish to know a person, we ask, What is their story, their real story? Each of us is a biography, a story. Stories are about what illness means to the individual and how that individual perceives the events that are occurring.
>
> (Sacks, 1983)

Brody (2003) argues that patients are most likely to improve when the meanings of their illness experience are altered in positive directions, when things are explained to them, when they feel cared for and when they achieve an enhanced degree of control over their lives. The greatest threat to patient recovery is the paternalistic health worker, who would, if not reined in, take all decision-making away from patients. Brody invites forensic mental health care workers to get close to clients emotionally and spiritually in order to understand them. It is in being understood that the first seedlings of healing and recovery can take root. We need to know much more about the experiences of forensic patients, more about the precursors of violent behaviours, why some reject before they are rejected and the types of help that people have found useful in their recovery (Wenzel, 2002).

In the 1990s, inadequacies in both the prison and health systems prompted a joint committee of the Home Office and the Health Service to be set up under the chairmanship of Dr John Reed. This was a landmark event in the history of forensic care in England (Snowden and Freeman, 1999). The subsequent Report identified, for the first time, guiding principles for the treatment of mentally disordered offenders, which were based on the needs of people rather than the protection of society.

GUIDING PRINCIPLES FOR THE CARE OF MENTALLY DISORDERED OFFENDERS

- High-quality care and proper attention should be given to the needs of individuals.
- Individuals should be cared for in the community rather than in institutions.
- No greater security should be present than is justified by the degree of risk that individuals present to others.
- Every assistance should be afforded to individuals through rehabilitation to increase their chances of sustaining an independent life.
- People should be cared for as close to their own homes and families as possible.

In order to achieve effective multidisciplinary working in forensic care, clarification of the role of forensic services is required, and of the roles of various professional groups. Improved collaboration between professional groups, and between professionals and other agencies is also needed (Konrad, 2002). Greater awareness of the influence of outside factors on forensic care is important. We should seek to gain more understanding of the widespread criminalisation of mentally ill people, economic constraints on treatment, the inadequacy of complementary, community-based care structures and the reluctance of general mental health services to accept mentally disordered offenders on the assumption that they pose a danger. There is also a pressing need to address the widespread disparity between teams, their composition and how they function and the problem of recruiting people to work in forensic services.

This chapter has attempted to provide a critical account of the development of and challenges facing forensic mental health care, while at the same time recognising and applauding what has been achieved in the care and treatment of people who require such services. Other chapters in this book will detail these achievements and demonstrate the progress that has been made towards multidisciplinary collaboration. Further study and research are required to determine more clearly what forensic services are for and who the beneficiaries should be. These thorny issues need to be tackled by all the disciplines involved, through conjoint working and thinking, in order that real progress can be made. Perhaps the greatest achievement might be to create forensic services where patients are cared for by personnel who create conditions where genuine inquiry can take place, where people are professional but curious and open to new ideas, where there is real commitment to respecting individuals and where improvement takes precedence over punishment and security. What is excellent in health care is invariably the result of the efforts not of any single discipline but of the many collaborating together.

References

Alderidge P (1979) Hospitals, madhouses, and asylums: cycles in the care of the insane. British Journal of Psychiatry 34: 321–334

Andrews J (1997) A failure to flourish? David Yellowlees and the Glasgow School of Psychiatry, Part 2. History of Psychiatry 8: 333–360

Applebaum P S (1997) A theory of ethics in forensic psychiatry. Journal of Academic Psychiatry Law 25: 233–247

Baum A and Dougall A (2002) Terrorism and behavioural medicine. Current Opinion in Psychiatry 15: 617–621

Bean P (1985) Social control and social theory in secure accommodation. In: Gostin L (ed.) Secure provision. London: Tavistock Publications

Berrios G A (1996) The history of mental symptoms. Cambridge: Cambridge University Press

Black J (1990) Eighteenth Europe. London: Macmillan

Bluglass R (1985) The development of regional secure units. In: Gostin L (ed.) Secure provision. London: Tavistock Publications

Bowden P (1991) Pioneers in forensic psychiatry; the acceptable face of psychiatry. Journal of Forensic Psychiatry 2: 59–78

Bowers L, Jarrett M, Clark N, Kiyimba F and McFarlane L (1999) 1. Absconding: why patients leave. Journal of Psychiatric and Mental Health Nursing 6(3): 199–206

Brody H (2003) Stories of sickness. Oxford: Oxford University Press

Campbell M, Fitzpatrick R and Haines A (2000) Framework for design and evaluation of complex interventions to improve health. British Medical Journal 321: 694–696

Carpenter M (2000) It's a small world: mental health policy under welfare capitalism since 1945. Sociology of Health and Illness 22: 602–620

Carpenter P (1989) Thomas Arnold; a provincial psychiatrist in Georgian England. Medical History 33: 199–216

Carpenter P (1997) The pauper insane of Leicester in 1844. History of Psychiatry 8: 517–537

Clarke B (1975) Mental disorder in early Britain. Cardiff: University of Wales Press

Coffey M and Jenkins E (2002) Power and control: forensic community mental health nurses' perceptions of team-working, legal sanction and compliance. Journal of Psychiatric and Mental Health Nursing 9: 521–529

Conacher N (1993) Issues in psychiatric care within a prison service. Canada's Mental Health 41: 11–15

Corrigan P W and McCracken S (1995) Psychiatric rehabilitation and staff development: educational and organisational models. Clinical Psychology Review 15: 699–719

Dingwall R, Rafferty A M and Webster C (1988) An introduction to the social history of nursing. London: Routledge

Gove D and Georges J (2001) Perspectives on legislation relating to the rights and protection of people with dementia in Europe. Aging Mental Health 5: 316–321

Gunn J (2000) Future directions for treatment in forensic psychiatry. British Journal of Psychiatry 176: 332–338

Halpern A L and Freedman A M (2002) Participation by physicians in legal executions in the USA: an update. Current Opinion in Psychiatry 15: 605–609

Hamilton J R (1985) The special hospitals. In: Gostin L (ed.) Secure provision. London: Tavistock Publications

Hogg M A and Vaughan G M (1995) Social psychology. London: Prentice Hall

International Association of Forensic Nurses (1999) Scope and standards of forensic practice. Washington: American Nurses Publishing

Knowles J (2003) Care and treatment under the Mental Health Act 1983. Nursing Times 99: 30–32

Konrad N (2002) Prisons as new asylums. Current Opinion in Psychiatry 15: 583–587

Lonsdale K (2001) The legal nurse consultant's role in forensic nursing. Journal of Legal Nurse Consultants 12: 17–20

Mason T (2002) Forensic psychiatric nursing: a literature review and thematic analysis of role tensions. Journal of Psychiatric and Mental Health Nursing 9: 511–520

Mercer D, Mason T, McKeown M and McCann G (eds) (2000) Forensic mental health care: a case study approach. London: Churchill Livingstone

Morrison E (1990) The tradition of toughness: a study of non-professional nursing care in psychiatric settings. Image: Journal of Nursing Scholarship 22: 32–38

Nettleton S (1995) The sociology of health and illness. London: Polity Press

Nolan P, Dallender J, Soares J and Arnetz B (1999) Violence in mental health care: the experience of mental health nurses and psychiatrists. Journal of Advanced Nursing 30: 934–941

O'Donoghue E G (1914) The Story of Bethlem Hospital. London: T. Fisher Unwin

Parker E (1985) The development of secure provision. In: Gostin L (ed.) Secure provision. London: Tavistock Publications

Porter R (1987) Mind forg'd manacles: madness and psychiatry in England from restoration to regency. London: Athlone Press

Porter R (1995) The eighteenth century. In: Lawrence I, Neave M, Nutton V, Porter R and Weir A (eds) The western tradition. Cambridge: Cambridge University Press

Porter R (2002) Madness, a brief history. Oxford: Oxford University Press

Prior P M (1997) Mad, not bad: crime, mental disorder and gender in nineteenth-century Ireland. History of Psychiatry 8: 501–516

Robinson A D (1988) A century of delusion in south west Scotland. British Journal of Psychiatry 153: 163–167

Sacks O (1983) Awakenings. New York: Dutton

Scull A (1977) Decarceration: community treatment and the deviant. New York: Prentice-Hall

Sedgwick P (1982) Psycho politics. London: Pluto Press

Skultans V (1979) English madness. London: Routledge and Kegan Paul

Smith L (1999) Cure, comfort and safe custody. Leicester: Leicester University Press

Smith R (1981) Trial by medicine: insanity and responsibility in Victorian trials. Edinburgh: Edinburgh University Press

Snowden P and Freeman H (1999) Forensic psychiatry. In: Freeman H (ed.) A century of psychiatry. London: Mosby–Wolfe

Stone A A (1994) Revisiting the parable: truth without consequences. International Journal of Law and Psychiatry 17: 79–97

Stone K (1997) The body political. London: Pluto

Taborda J G and Abdalla-Filho E (2002) Ethics in forensic psychiatry. Current Opinion in Psychiatry 15: 599–603

Tajfel H and Turner J C (1979) An integrative theory of inter-group conflict. In: Austin WG and Worchel S (eds) The social psychology of inter-group relations. Monterey: CA Brooks/Cole

Thompson P (1972) Bound for Broadmoor. London: Hodder and Stoughton

Thomsen S, Soares J, Nolan P, Dallender J and Arnetz B (1999) Feelings of professional fulfilment and exhaustion in mental health personnel: the importance of organisational and individual factors. Psychotherapy and Psychosomatics 68: 157–164

Turner B S (1987) Medical power and social knowledge. London: Sage

Unsworth C (1987) The politics of mental health legislation. Oxford: Clarendon Press

Wenzel T (2002) Forensic evaluation of sequels to torture. Current Opinion in Psychiatry 15: 611–615

Woods C (2002) Guest editorial. Journal of Psychiatric and Mental Health Nursing 9: 492–494

Chapter 2

Theoretical foundation

Rebecca A. Hills

INTRODUCTION

The health team has been defined as 'a group who share common health goals and common objectives, determined by community needs, to the achievement of which each member contributes, in accordance with his or her competence and skill and in coordination with the functions of others' (WHO, 1984: 13). Over the years, health care has constantly changed and developed; throughout this ongoing shift in practice and focus, trends have and will continue to emerge. One such trend has been the emergence of interprofessional working both as a practice and a concept. There are whole ranges of pressures upon those who provide health and social care that have prompted the development of interprofessional and interagency working. The way that health services are organised and managed has also affected the delivery of care. Rodgers (1994) argues that the development of the internal market in the National Health Service resulted in collaborative practice becoming essential. Investigation of the subject of 'interprofessional working' presents the reader with a complicated selection of terminology often with the same or similar meaning. Leathard (1994) divided the most commonly used alternative phrases into those that are *concept based*, those that are *process based* and those that are *agency based* (Leathard, 1994: 5). Examples of concept-based terms are perhaps the best-known—'multidisciplinary', 'multiprofessional' and 'generic'. Process-based terms are, for example, 'collaboration', 'integration' and 'teamwork', and those that are agency based include 'interagency' and 'intersectoral'. The value of working in multiprofessional or interprofessional teams will be discussed later in this chapter. However, when developing teams and team working practice, it is important to remember that there is limited evidence to demonstrate that team working improves the quality of care provided to the user of the service. The question of why interprofessional working should be used within forensic mental health can most easily be answered by an examination of mental health inquiry reports published in Britain over the last decade. Careful consideration of these reports highlights the elements of team working, interprofessional working or multidisciplinary working that are essential when working with individuals who have complex mental health and social needs.

Suffolk Health Authority (1996) examined the case of Jason Mitchell, who killed three people while being treated by mental health services and having been made the subject of a hospital order with restrictions (section 37/41) of the Mental Health Act 1983. Within their report, a number of relevant comments are made. The report states (Suffolk Health Authority, 1996: 273) that 'lack of teamwork between medical and non-medical professionals was never more apparent (than at a specific stage in the case)'. The report questions lack of referrals to others, which appeared to be required, but were not made thus demonstrating both poor interprofessional and poor interagency practice. One of the most definite points made within the report is that all team members must be regarded as essential, therefore, any information they pass on to the team must be considered valid. The panel also commented on several aspects of communication within teams: they suggested that contributions from team members other than nurses and doctors should be systematically recorded within all relevant records.

Likewise, Blom Cooper et al. (1995) reported on the killing of Georgina Robinson, an occupational therapist who was killed by Andrew Robinson, a patient at Torbay District Hospital. Within the report of the inquiry into the case, the inability for single professions to provide the level of input needed by individuals using mental health services is highlighted: 'to address the diversity of needs thrown up in the person with severe mental illness is a daunting task for any well integrated and coordinated team. For any single professional it is well nigh impossible' (Blom Cooper et al., 1995: 135). Again, in this report, the authors concur with others that a clear understanding of the roles and responsibilities of all team members, and high-quality communication is essential. In addition, the report into this incident identifies the need for clear and consistent boundaries when working with patients who have severe mental health problems. This, the report suggests, is an aspect of care that can only be achieved effectively by the collaboration and consultation that multidisciplinary team working provides.

Sheppard (1996) summarises selected recommendations made by inquiries published between 1985 and 1996. In this he notes 80 recommendations that are related to multidisciplinary or interagency working. Many of these are recommendations about methods of communication; however, they also cover roles within the team, training needs, accountability within the team and the resolution of disagreements about the clinical care of patients. This summary would seem to offer a valuable reflection of what are considered to be the central issues to team working generally. This chapter will further consider why health and social care professionals aim towards working successfully and effectively in teams. It will outline models of teamwork and discuss roles, language used and leadership.

FOUNDATIONS—WHY WORK IN TEAMS?

The dictionary definition of the word 'team' provides us with an initial and perhaps somewhat superficial answer to this question—'a group of people organised to work together' (Collins Concise English Dictionary, 1991: 1030). However, it is important to keep this simplistic view in mind when considering the question 'why', as it provides us with the framework within which to identify the more complex reasons why working in teams is considered the ideal within current health care provision. Leiba (1994: 137) says that 'interprofessional teamwork is neither a good nor a bad thing; it is an unavoidable social construction in mental health services, where the contributions and professional expertise of each worker are called for if citizens are to obtain the services they need in a coordinated way'. If this is so, the development of the team may be viewed as somewhat inevitable: simply a method of operating services, upon which the professions and, indeed, the client has little, if any, control. Sociologists describe social groups as being effectively either 'primary' or 'secondary' (Goodman, 1992), the primary social group being a small group that provides the individual with close and long-lasting relationships. These are groups, such as families, where the group have shared experiences and history, and may spend or have spent considerable time together. Secondary social groups, however, are by definition temporary groups, which are established to achieve a specific purpose and which operate while the shared purpose remains, but which have limited long-term impact on the members of the group. Goodman (1992) notes, however, that it is possible for the secondary groups that remain together for extensive periods of time to begin to take on some of the characteristics of the primary group, such as sharing confidences, carrying out daily routines (e.g. having lunch) together and getting to know each other better outside of the work focus of the team. The central difference between these types of group is the 'emotional investment in the group and in each other' (Goodman, 1992: 58). It could be argued that health care teams, although taking the role of a secondary social group when established, frequently become primary social groups as they develop and extend their role in the individual member's work life.

The development of the use of health and social care teams, and now integrated care teams may be due to a response to a wide range of social and economic issues. Kane (1980) describes team working developing within social work in response to a relative lack of power. She recognised this developing (since the 1970s) in the other professions, initially nursing, pharmacy and occupational therapy, and eventually, although more latterly, in the medical profession. The desire of these professions, it seems, was to be able to offer a more coordinated and, therefore, more effective service to the client group. McGrath (1991) reasons that health and social care workers need to work in teams for two central reasons: to ensure effective service provision, and to produce a more satisfying working environment. She argues that the multiprofessional team provides a holistic approach to client needs, allows system problems to be tackled and encourages overall service planning and preventative work. However, the perception that the use of teams in health and social care is always of value to the client must also be questioned. Webb and Hobdell (1980: 98), for example, are critical of British social work, saying that the profession misdirected its energy 'in search of the holy grail of interprofessional collaboration', instead of increasing its specialist skills, which is what, they suggest, is needed by the client. They conclude that it would be foolish to assume that teamwork and improved client care are synonymous. For the individual worker, the benefit of working as a member of a team may be, as sociology describes, the achievement of a common purpose, the completion of a task and in well-established longer-term teams, the development of emotional bonds between the team members. However, there are also associated issues, such as those of pay and status differentials, for the individual working in a team which may be fraught with difficulty.

In order that the interprofessional team works effectively, it is necessary to recognise that there are also inevitable barriers. Leiba (1996) quotes Strauss (1962), who argued that professionalism in itself is a barrier to team and collaborative working. The features that create a profession, that is, specialist opinions, underpinning philosophy and a particular view of the world, are also the aspects that produce barriers to working together. It is, therefore, the development of clinical care goals to which each profession can contribute that will overcome such barriers (Leiba, 1996). Professional beliefs firmly held by the individual practitioner are established within the professional training. It is the development of professional skills and values during training on 'segregated courses and sometimes in separate institutions' (Leiba, 1996: 137) that limits the individual's ability to understand the roles of other professionals within the team, and consequently creates barriers to communication and effective collaborative working as team members. However, the development of many training courses with at least shared core modules is at least going some way towards addressing this. Leiba also cites the 'divided loyalties' of many of the team members as a barrier to successful (or enjoyable) team working. The development of general management within health care, and the integration of health and social care teams have left many practitioners with dual accountability within parallel structures. Many staff will be part of a line management within the team or service for 'operational' issues; they will also be professionally accountable within the relevant professional hierarchy. Although when working well they are tools for truly integrative practice, these structures depend upon well-established and agreed systems for managing contradictive instruction or advice to the practitioner.

It must be remembered that there are definite disadvantages to teamwork. McGrath (1991) suggests that these are the time it takes to consult adequately, the accountability to peers, which is felt by some p... ers to be threatening, and the conflict in loyalties as defined abov... Jones (1986: 193) also cautions against unquestioning accept...ce of multiprofessional team working in mental health, where he says history clearly shows the pitfalls of not closely examining any approach adopted. He reminds us that team working practice must be closely scrutinised to ensure it is the most efficient and effective method of providing care. However, he also points out that, in the area he is reviewing (adolescent mental health), 'no single group, service or agency has the capacity to manage all aspects of all cases', a statement that could certainly be equally true of forensic mental health.

MODELS OF TEAM WORKING

Health and social care practitioners readily describe themselves as working in a 'team'. Although most workers would rarely consider the model of teamwork in which they are working, the practice in itself appears to have become embedded in most areas of health and social care. 'Multiprofessional', 'multidisciplinary' or 'interprofessional' teamwork has become the model of practice preferred and 'promoted for many areas of health care by policy makers, professional bodies and Trust management' (Freeman et al., 2000: 237). The underlying belief to the adoption of this model being; as discussed in a previous section, that working in teams improves the care provided to service users.

Freeman et al. (2000) identified three interpretations of team working using evidence gained from six case studies. Within the study they looked at teams operating in a range of clinical fields, including a diabetes team and community mental health team. They note that, although the individual philosophies that they identified were in some cases relevant to the profession of the practitioner, this was not always the case. The philosophies that the study identified are detailed below.

Directive

This was related strongly to the team members' beliefs about status and hierarchy. It is described as being held most frequently by members of the medical profession. It has relevance to the levels of communication used within the team—the 'team leader' determines 'what, when and how communication was communicated and to whom' (Freeman et al., 2000: 241). Teams working within this philosophy were also characterised by those at higher levels in the hierarchy believing they had little or nothing to learn from those at more junior levels in the structure; junior workers were also valued more for what they offered to the more powerful roles than for what they offered to the care of the service user. This philosophy may invariably resonate with some aspects of forensic mental health care. The status of the most senior medical member of the team as 'responsible medical officer' (RMO) under the Mental Health Act 1983 immediately produces a variation in status both within the team and in terms of interaction with the Criminal Justice System. The RMO is almost inevitably the team leader in practice, if not always in name. Anecdotally, it is not unusual for the team to be called or known by the

RMO's surname (hence a team with Dr Smith as RMO would be known locally as 'the Smith team').

Integrative

This philosophy is identified as being one in which the team members demonstrated commitment to two aspects: the practice of collaborative care and therapy, and a recognition of 'Different levels of role understanding and their importance in the development of negotiated role boundaries' (Freeman et al., 2000: 241). This philosophy was also characterised by the use of discussion and negotiation in the development of the understanding of the needs of the service user; unlike the directive philosophy, it also meant that there is a belief that each team member can learn from other members. This philosophy may be more easily identifiable in specialist teams working within the field of forensic mental health. Within such teams, a shared level or expectation of 'expertise' may be more apparent and the role of RMO less dominant. Examples may be specialist sex-offender teams, where members of a wide variety of agencies are considered both expert and of equal value (an example might be a team coordinated by a clinical psychologist but with members from probation, the Home Office, social services and the police).

Elective

This philosophy was described as 'essentially a system of liaison' (Freeman et al., 2000: 241). It describes those professionals who operated autonomously from the other professionals involved in the care of the service user. Communication was maintained but was characterised by its 'brevity'. This philosophy also maintained the hierarchical nature of the directive philosophy as described. It is possible to identify specific groups within forensic mental health who continue to work with at least partial autonomy. Different services may be able to identify different groups to which this philosophy may apply; this may be due to the organisation of practice or the role beliefs of the particular professional, examples of which may be complementary therapists or teaching staff within some organisations.

Rawson (1994) considers models of team working in the terms of 'implied mathematics'. Within this framework he describes two versions of interprofessional work that are possible. These are the *additive model* (Rawson, 1994: 41), whereby each member profession adds its own expertise and perspective, the professions are considered of equal value and importance and all contributions are taken into account. The *multiplicative model*, however, enables the team to achieve more than is possible than by simply joining all the professions together. Here interprofessional working in itself promotes initiative and innovation, and Rawson describes it as 'more than the sum of its parts'.

Rawson (1994: 43) considers the aim of many organisations to achieve what is termed 'seamless' services as being suggestive of the 'dissolution of boundaries'. He describes this as allowing the transfer of 'elements' across 'sets' or professional groupings. This could be viewed as the sharing of specific skills and perhaps the development of what have become known as 'generic' skills. Thus, the professions maintain their differences only within their own core skills. Rawson further develops this by acknowledging that those professional groups working together with 'mutually impermeable' boundaries must reach agreements, which are mutually agreeable—this model he titles the *mutual respect model.*

Finally Rawson describes what he titles the *melting pot model.* Within this model, the team's needs and goals supersede those defined by the original occupational groupings. The team becomes similar in practice and function to a profession in its own right.

Forensic mental health demonstrates a range of models of teamwork that vary across services and to some extent within services. Examples of all the models described can be found within the clinical field. An understanding of how the team practices and the influences upon it allow the practitioner to identify the skills needed to operate effectively within it.

ISSUES

The multidisciplinary team may be made up of a range of disciplines, working in a whole variety of settings even within the specialist field of forensic mental health. Each team may appear very different from one another; however, it is likely that they will all, almost certainly, face several issues, which can be categorised into *goal related, role related, procedural, problem solving or interpersonal* (Rubin and Bechard, 1979; cited in Engel, 1994: 66). *Goal-related issues* refer to those issues about identifying the team's goal and, therefore, the related objectives. The goal within forensic mental health may often appear to be relatively straightforward. The primary goal of most aspects of the service may be to ensure that the individual is assessed and treated, while the potential risk to the individual and the wider community is managed safely and effectively. However, within this primary goal, it can be seen that each discipline or indeed practitioner may prioritise certain aspects over others.

Role-related issues

These are issues that arise from 'the need to articulate and resolve any differences in what members expect from one another in their day to day performance and behaviour' (Engel, 1994: 66). This may be difficult within particular teams within any specialist clinical area. In forensic mental health status within the team often varies enormously. The variation in status or perceived status can inhibit the ability of practitioners who occupy different positions in the hierarchy to resolve differences, or to challenge one another on aspects of performance or behaviour.

Procedural issues

These are essentially issues around 'procedure' with regard to decision-making and, therefore, accountability. This is again an area that has particular relevance to forensic mental health teams. Decisions in such teams, as in many clinical areas, carry with them significant risk. The responsible medical officer (consultant psychiatrist) carries the weight of accountability for clinical decisions made by the team. This position may lead to other members of the team feeling that 'shared' decision-making is an illusion. It should be remembered, however, that all registered health and social care practitioners are accountable for their own actions.

Problem–solving issues

These are issues that arise from the need to resolve difficulties. The solving of problems or difficulties is an essential component of team working. The aspect that is often absent, however, is an agreed method for how this should be done.

Interpersonal issues

This refers to those issues that arise out of the relationships that are established within the team and the way in which team members interact. As in any group of people, these issues can take an infinite variety of forms. They will relate to the very different personalities who work within the team.

ROLES

The influence of professional role and the perception of other members of the team are well established as a critical aspect of team working. Although Rawson (1994: 49) suggests that the concept of 'role' is possibly overused in consideration of interprofessional work, we are reminded that the term 'role' refers to 'the functions of a position within the structure of a group'. It is essential, for the purpose of interprofessional work, that there is a difference between the position of each professional group within the team, which specifies task characteristics and how professional perspective affects the way the job is shaped. Rawson describes how roles are most noteworthy in research terms when they are related to conflict within the structure.

However, on an operational level, the lack of knowledge that health and social care practitioners have about one another's role within the multidisciplinary team has been noted. Milne (1981) studied this aspect of teamwork within a group of health care students. The study demonstrated a pattern that Milne described as 'role enquiry' during which members were surprised by their own lack of knowledge about what others do, and 'role uncertainty' in which members of like professions were seen to have incongruent opinions. McGee and Ashford (1996) also studied role perception within multidisciplinary teams. They concluded that, in order that a genuine understanding of the role of others in the team is developed, shared teaching at undergraduate level is essential. Herrman et al. (2002) described obstacles to effective teamwork being, amongst other components, ambiguity and conflict over roles alongside interprofessional misperceptions.

They describe the tension between 'team member's desire for clarity of roles and the need for flexibility' (Herrman et al., 2002: 76). Peck and Norman (1999) reported on a study that was established to examine problems of interprofessional working in adult community mental health. It was identified that team members experienced problems in being able to establish and sustain a system of effective collaboration

across disciplines. They concluded that this was 'relate~
ferences in culture between professional groups and to the ~
ues held by group members' (Peck and Norman, 1999: 231). The ~
demonstrated the value of 'promoting understanding of professional
roles' as a method of promoting interprofessional collaboration.

Within the specialist area of forensic mental health, the nurse within
the team is often considered the most crucial member of the team, particularly within inpatient services. The nursing group often constitutes
the largest group by some considerable margin within such services. It is
essential, therefore, that the nurses themselves, the patient group and the
rest of the interprofessional team have a clear and realistic view of the
nursing role. Dale and Tarbuck (1995) examined the role of the nurse
within a high security hospital (Ashworth in Merseyside) to consider
some of the difficulties facing nursing following a public inquiry at the
hospital in 1992 that had commented on the denigrating culture that
existed at Ashworth. They described how 'we found that nurses and
patients were in such similar situations that both could be described as
victims' (Peck and Norman, 1995: 33). The authors describe the conflict-
ing pressures facing nurses within this environment, where they are
caught between their professional ethics, which drive them to empower
and support the patients in their care and their role within society, which
is to 'control' patients and protect the wider community from harm. A
similar argument regarding the role of the nurse within secure environments is made by Mason and Chandley (1990). They too identify the
fundamental difficulty for nurses of operating in a system where they
serve the dual role of nurse and 'guard'. They conclude that these difficulties face nursing within secure environments as a direct result of the
'medicalisation of criminology'. However, alongside these specific issues
for nursing within the forensic mental health field, the role and scope of
nursing is developing in the wider context. Clinical nurse specialist roles
are now well established and the more recent development of nurse consultant posts across many areas of health care, including forensic mental
health, has promoted nurses ostensibly to a similar status as their colleagues in medicine and psychology.

The NHS Plan (Department of Health, 2000) included provision for
similar roles in occupational therapy. The behaviour that professionals or
'subcultures' within health care demonstrate is part of the ritual that
maintains their position within the service and hierarchy (Brooks and
Brown, 2002). This is an important element of team working behaviour
to consider when identifying roles and the development of shared working. The increase in genericism has presented health professionals with
many dilemmas as the behaviours, which are historically attached to
their professional roles, are eroded. The identification of the core skills of
each profession also enables the team worker to clarify those tasks that
can realistically and safely be carried out by any team member. Brooks
and Brown (2002: 341) describe two bands of 'ceremonial' behaviour that
are related to this: those which 'preserve the existing norms and autonomy of professional groups' and those which 'encourage change'. The
constant shifting sands of role and role development within the broad

area of health and social care and, more specifically, within mental health require ongoing and scrupulous investigation in order that the most effective and appropriate systems of collaborative team working are developed. Masterson (2002) describes work by McCoy in which 'service developments and policy initiatives interact in a mutually reinforcing way to create and maintain the illusion of success without recourse to empirical evidence'. It is essential that the impact of role and the perception of role as inhibitors or promoters of effective team working are viewed as valuable areas for research and development.

LANGUAGE AND COMMUNICATION

Pietroni (1992) describes the 'baby' of interprofessional work that is hindered by the need to develop a language, which can be shared by all its members. This is a description that will surely resonate with most health and social care staff as well as workers from the many agencies with which they communicate and collaborate. Pietroni classifies the languages of disciplines being from one of 11 philosophical bases (such as medical, psychological, social, economic and environmental), which he says forms the foundations of the language that disciplines or professions devise to describe or define their view of the world. This, he says, is why practitioners who are essentially formed from different philosophical bases have such difficulty talking to and understanding one another. Following this view through to its conclusion, Pietroni recommends that rather than trying to change one another's language, we should actually attempt to integrate the language subsets that currently exist using reflective practice within the team. The rudiments of these negotiations often take place during team-building days, but it seems of great importance to acknowledge that this is what is happening, as the use of 'interpretable' language can effectively make or break a team (Pietroni, 1992). However, in order for reflective practitioners to be able to develop their skills at communicating their own language and, therefore, values to those of other professions, they need to be clear about their values themselves. This requires a certain degree of professional maturity and flexibility from the practitioner (Wilmot, 1995). Within forensic mental health, communication, as a part of interprofessional working, has been demonstrated time and again to be essential. Sheppard (1996) summarises selected recommendations made by inquiries published between 1985 and 1996. In this he notes 80 recommendations, which are related to multidisciplinary or multiagency working. Many of these are about methods of communication.

The issue of hierarchy has a clear impact on the use and value of interprofessional communication within the team. Engstrom (1986) describes the hierarchy within the health care team in which the doctor and nurse occupy noticeably different positions. It is noted that, as a result of the differing hierarchical positions, the doctors within meetings such as case conferences have a tendency to become overloaded with medical information and, therefore, put far less emphasis on sociopsychological factors. If this is not managed carefully by both the doctor and the rest of the team, it may result in the patients not receiving the information they need in order to make both an informed decision and to take an active role in their care. This is perhaps another issue that may be best resolved within regular team reflective practice meetings. The role of the chairperson is essential if the impact of hierarchy is not to distract from the focus of the team. Chairing such meetings can be extremely challenging and can be impacted upon by the hierarchy in itself; members of the team who are to take on this role should be provided with the opportunity to prepare for the role and to develop the skills in the same way as any other professional skill is developed. Engstrom (1986: 301) describes how the chairperson has 'an important role in mastering the difficulties which lie in all possibilities for erroneous interpretation and misunderstandings which can occur in a communication process in which several individuals are involved'.

At a basic level, one of the most fundamental differences between disciplines and agencies is the title of the 'subject' of their work. Hornby (1993) illustrates this clearly with her script of a meeting of a variety of different practitioners in which the meeting attendees refer variously to their 'client', 'pupil' and 'patient'. This is difference in language and difficulty in communication at its most fundamental, and potentially at its most damaging. However, within the world of forensic mental health, it is a situation that happens frequently. The need for practitioners to work both with other health disciplines, other social care disciplines but also probation, the police, the Crown Prosecution Service, lawyers, the prison service and the Home Office amongst others is essential. The need to be clear about what is being said about the service user, to whom and who has responsibility for which task is vital in order that the dual aims of treating the service user whilst also maintaining the safety of the community, within legal and ethical boundaries, are met.

Opportunities for the health and social care professions to improve their ability to understand each other and, therefore, to communicate more effectively with one another with an aim to developing collaborative practice can be seen as the key to improved forensic mental health services. There is a vast amount of literature available that examines these opportunities. The development of shared training and education programmes is one of the most basic of these opportunities. It is within undergraduate and pre-registration courses that practitioners learn their professional language and the behaviour that is associated with it. It is at this level that practitioners are able to absorb the differences between the professions without the associations that they develop in later practice. Many undergraduate and postgraduate courses are now developing core modules in which all or many of the professions training in the institution will participate. The experience of learning alongside members of another profession is invaluable in breaking down the communication barriers. Integrated services and joint planning of services demands 'joint finance mechanisms as well as the development of cooperative strategies' (Owens et al., 1995: 151). However, shared strategy in which the goals of each agency are explicit promotes the level of collaboration needed at the grass roots of the operation. An example of such a combined strategy was established in Surrey (Haynes and Henfrey, 1995: 4).

The authors of the report about the strategy note 'the willingness of the criminal justice players to learn the language of the community care policy process and internal market was crucial'. At a more local level, shared business plans, in which each department or discipline jointly subscribes to shared goals, provides a framework within which the practitioner can operate effectively. Finally, the use of the Care Programme Approach (Department of Health, 1990) should enforce communication and collaborative practice. If used as it should be, the role of the care coordinator, who may be from any discipline, enforces cross-disciplinary working and demands a certain level of understanding of one another's roles and responsibilities.

LEADERSHIP

Kenneth Calman, in a lecture in 1994, said that all teams need leaders as 'they need heroes who by vision and hard work take the team forward' (Calman, 1994: 97). Team working invariably involves members of the team taking on roles within the group. Each role serves a purpose both for the team and for the team member themselves. The role that potentially has a great impact on the other members of the team and on the work of the team itself is that of team leader. Within forensic mental health, as within many health care teams, there may be more than one leader. There may be either an administrative leader or manager, and there may be the member of the team who has the greatest level of clinical accountability. There may also be a focus towards a particular role as 'leader', owing to historical or hierarchical issues. In forensic mental health, the leader of the interprofessional team is most frequently the consultant psychiatrist who has the legal responsibilities of the responsible medical officer role. Sociologists describe groups as having leaders who are those 'who by virtue of personality, accomplishments or position play a major role in affecting the activities of the group' (Goodman, 1992: 64).

Leadership has two main functions, and leaders may demonstrate skills in carrying out either or both of these functions. The instrumental or task-orientated leader works towards the group identifying, planning or completing a task, thereby achieving the common objective of the group, while the expressive or relationship-orientated leader is concerned with the well-being of the group itself. In order for the group or team to be at its most effective, elements of both styles are necessary. Blake and Mouton (1964) defined leadership styles as being characterised by varying levels or 'dimensions' across the spectrum of task or relationship focus (Maslin, 1991). Therefore, the leader may be high relationship and low task, high task and high relationship, low relationship and low task or high task and low relationship in their style or type of leadership. Sociology also describes leadership styles as being 'democratic', 'authoritarian' or 'laissez faire' (Goodman, 1992). Leadership has two main functions, and leaders may demonstrate skills in carrying out either in isolation or by combining both these functions.

Engel (1994) views the role of the team leader as a great challenge. He describes the role of the leader as primarily to 'facilitate their team's collaboration as it focuses on the client, the patient, the carer or the family' (Engel, 1994: 68). He also reminds us not to forget their role as ambassador or diplomat. The difficulty for the leader of a team within forensic mental health may be trying to lead a team that has loyalties to a variety of other bodies or groups. Frequently team members in these settings also have membership of a team within their own profession, of management teams or of other specialist teams within the service. They may (in the case of social work) be employed by a different organisation than other team members and have loyalty to that organisation. Similar issues are described by Mason et al. (2002) when describing a 'three-level ethical code of reference' used by staff in forensic mental health teams. These were identified as: (a) within their individual ideological framework; (b) reference to the local unit or Trust; and (c) reference to the professional code to which they belonged (Mason et al., 2002: 569). These variations in terms of reference and in loyalties or degree of belonging present the leader with a very specific challenge—that of ensuring that team members are working within compatible frames of reference and are feeling valued enough within the team to produce collaborative practice, which meets the needs of the patient group.

It is vital for effective interprofessional teamwork that accountability and responsibility are discussed, identified and acknowledged by all the members of the team. Within forensic mental health teams, this can raise a number of issues for team members, which may affect their practice. Griffin (1989) describes an approach that attaches 'full clinical responsibility' to the consultant psychiatrist in the role of responsible medical officer. This acknowledges the legal responsibility that is attached to this role. At present, the consultant psychiatrist is the only member of the team who carries this responsibility, although it could be envisaged that this is a role that could be adopted by others in specific clinical areas in the future; an example being a consultant psychologist in the care of individuals with personality disorder. However, Griffin also attaches 'independent professional responsibility' to each member of the team. All health and social care practitioners work within a code of practice, which is usually defined by their professional body; for many professions, their registration remains dependent on their accepting the responsibility that being a registered practitioner puts upon them. The essential ingredient to team working is often considered the level of responsibility that each member of the team takes for the decisions made by the team and, therefore, the sharing of responsibility for the outcome of those decisions. This may be the hardest task that the team leader has to achieve.

CONCLUSION

The need for professionals working in every field of health and social care is considered indisputable. The care of the mentally disordered offender within the services provided by forensic mental health services may be considered to present the case for interprofessional working in its most extreme form, as the consequences for the patient, the professional and the wider community are potentially devastating without it. The evidence for the value of team working in improving quality of care to the same patient group is somewhat limited, however. The presence of the term 'interprofessional' or 'multidisciplinary' in common health care terminology does not necessarily imply that collaborative practices are being carried out, still less that these represent the production of more effective patient care. It is essential that all health and social care professionals are given the opportunity to develop an understanding of the theory underlying teamwork, and to develop the skills required to work effectively within them. Kane (1980) described the three common elements present in teams as being shared aims, the presence of distinct roles for team members, and a structure to facilitate joint working and communication. These elements offer a yardstick by which teams are able to measure their potential for effectiveness.

References

Blake R and Mouton J (1964) The management grid. London: Gulf Publishing

Blom Cooper L, Hally H and Murphy E (1995) The falling shadow. London: Duckworth

Brooks I and Brown B (2002) The role of ritualistic ceremonial in removing barriers between subcultures in the National Health Service. Journal of Advanced Nursing 4: 341–352

Calman K (1994) Working together, teamwork. Journal of Interprofessional Care 1: 95–99

Collins Concise English Dictionary (1991) English dictionary, 2nd edn. Glasgow: Harper Collins Publishers

Dale C and Tarbuck P (1995) Changing the nursing culture in a special hospital. Nursing Times 30: 33–35

Department of Health (1990) The Care Programme Approach for people with mental illness referred to the specialist psychiatric services, DOH HC 90 23/LASL. London: HMSO

Department of Health (2000) The NHS Plan, A plan for investment a plan for reform. London: HMSO

Engel C (1994) A functional anatomy of teamwork. In Leathard A (ed.) Going interprofessional—working together for health and welfare. London: Routledge

Engstrom B (1986) Communication and decision making in a study of multidisciplinary team conference with the registered nurse as conference chairman. International Journal of Nursing Studies 4: 299–314

Freeman M, Miller C and Ross N (2000) The impact of individual philosophies of teamwork on multi-professional practice and the implications for education. Journal of Interprofessional Care 14: 3

Goodman N (1992) Introduction to sociology. London: Harper Collins

Griffin N (1989) Multi professional care in forensic psychiatry. Psychiatric Bulletin 13: 613–615

Haynes P and Henfrey D (1995) Progress in partnership and collaboration: an evaluation of multi-agency working for mentally disordered offenders in Surrey. University of Brighton

Herrman H, Trauer T and Warnock J (2002) The roles and relationships of psychiatrists and other service providers in mental health services. Australian and New Zealand Journal of Psychiatry 36: 75–80

Hornby S (1993) Collaborative care interagency, interprofessional, interpersonal. Oxford: Blackwell Scientific Publications

Kane R (1980) Multidisciplinary teamwork in the United States: trends, issues and implications for the social worker. In Lonsdale S, et al. (eds) Teamwork in personal social services and healthcare. London: Croom Helm

Leathard A (1994) Going inter-professional. Working together for health and welfare. London: Routledge

Leiba T (1994) Inter-professional approaches to mental health care. In Leathard A (ed.) Going interprofessional. London: Routledge

Leiba T (1996) Interprofessional and multi-agency training and working. British Journal of Community Health Nursing 1: 8–12

Maslin Z (1991) Management in occupational therapy. London: Chapman and Hall

Mason T and Chandley M (1990) Nursing models in a special hospital; a critical analysis of efficacy. Journal of Advanced Nursing 15: 667–673

Mason T, Williams R and Vivian-Byrne S (2002) Multidisciplinary working in a forensic mental health setting: ethical codes of reference. Journal of Psychiatric and Mental Health Nursing 9: 563–572

Masterson A (2002) Cross-boundary working: a macro political analysis of the impact on professional roles. Journal of Clinical Nursing 11: 331–339

McGee P and Ashford R (1996) Nurses' perceptions of roles in multi disciplinary teams. Nursing Standard 45: 34–36

McGrath M (1991) Multidisciplinary teamwork. Aldershot: Avebury

Milne M (1981) The primary healthcare team: linked group discussions as a learning medium. Journal of Advanced Nursing 6: 349–354

Owens P, Carrier J and Horder J (1995) Interprofessional issues in community and primary health care. London: Macmillan

Parry Jones W (1986) Multi disciplinary teamwork: help or hindrance? In Steinberg D (ed.) The adolescent unit—work and teamwork in adolescent psychiatry. Chichester: Wiley

Peck E and Norman I (1999) Working together in adult community mental health services: exploring interprofessional role relations. Journal of Mental Health 8: 231–242

Pietroni P (1992) Towards reflective practice—the languages of health and social care. Journal of Interprofessional Care 1: 7–16

Rawson D (1994) Models of interprofessional work. In Leathard A (ed.) Going interprofessional—working together for health and social care. London: Routledge

Rodgers J (1994) Collaboration among health professionals. Nursing Standard 6: 25–26

Sheppard D (1996) Learning the lessons. London: The Zito Trust

Suffolk Health Authority (1996) The case of Jason Mitchell: The report of the Panel of Inquiry. London: Duckworth

Webb A and Hobdell M (1980) Co-ordination and teamwork in the health and personal social services. In Lonsdale S et al. (eds) Teamwork in personal social services and healthcare: risk and response. London: Duckworth

Wilmot S (1995) Professional values and interprofessional dialogue. Journal of Interprofessional Care 9: 257–265

World Health Organization (1984) The role of WHO participating centers in continuing education, specialty training and educational research. Copenhagen: World Health Organisation

Chapter **3**

The multidisciplinary team and clinical team meetings

Martin Humphreys

INTRODUCTION

The theoretical basis and foundation of multidisciplinary working may be very different from the practical realities of the day-to-day demands placed on the team and its members. The individuals who make up the team almost invariably come from very different professional backgrounds but equally the composition of the team may change over time. There may be periods during which certain professions are not represented at all. In addition, for whatever reason, there may be different personnel coming and going from within one or more of the professional groups that make up the whole. At least as important for the day-to-day running of the team and the clinical practice of its members will be the personalities of the individuals who work in it, the team's history, the immediate working environment and the wider institution within which it is based. Likewise, the commitment of the team members to unified aims and objectives and the relative standing of each within the team itself, and also within their own individual professions, may have a major impact on its functioning. Resources, in terms of manpower and staffing, but also in what might seem superficially to be rather less important areas, such as working and office space, administrative support and access to appropriate levels of supervision for each of the individual members of the team, are also likely to have a major influence on morale and working practice.

The various training requirements for each of the constituent professions will differ and must be accounted for. The need to incorporate students from different disciplines into the team on occasions, sometimes for quite brief periods, as well as trainees on longer-term secondment or placement, will also inevitably affect the team dynamic. Additional professional commitments for individual team members outside its day-to-day functioning may equally alter the balance. Interpersonal interactions and alliances, and their nature and quality, between members of the team at a non-professional level, for instance, involvement in common outside interests, longstanding friendships, particularly close working, or even more intimate personal relationships, may also have a profound effect on the team's potential or actual functioning.

TEAM MEMBERSHIP

There is a descriptive caricature of a multidisciplinary forensic mental health team, which reads thus:

- The consultant forensic psychiatrist leads the team by absolute right, directs the junior medical staff to see patients and write prescriptions, and spends the remainder of his or her time writing long and complex, wordy legal reports for substantial fees, and waxing lyrical from the witness box.
- The clinical psychologist measures IQ and other things with exhaustive and intricate questionnaires that no one else is allowed to use and no one else understands anyway. He or she also explains the patient's offending behaviour in terms of attachment theory or transitional objects.
- The junior doctor sees patients and writes prescriptions as directed by the consultant.
- The senior nurse undertakes all assessments for admission, deals with most of the day-to-day running of the inpatient unit and calms everyone's nerves in a crisis.
- The social worker fills in claim forms and, in the case of conditionally discharged restricted patients, is, as social supervisor, the policeman of the state and the 'eyes and ears of the Home Office'.
- The forensic community psychiatric nurse (CPN) intrudes on people's lives on a regular basis by visiting them at home and injecting them with toxic medications.
- The occupational therapist supervises basket-weaving activities.
- The pharmacist counts pills.
- The team secretary runs the day-to-day business of managing team members and the team as a whole, runs meetings, keeps diaries, records clinical work and undertakes all the other necessary administrative tasks and knows immediately everything that anyone, from within the team or from the outside world, could possibly wish to know!

Of course, this is no more than a facetious characterisation, hopefully bearing little or no resemblance to real life. Nevertheless, there is a need for individuals working within a team structure in forensic mental health care, to have a clear understanding of the roles and abilities of their fellow team members, a degree of mutual respect and a willingness to offer support.

Multidisciplinary team membership in forensic mental health care settings will vary with time, the availability of human resources, recruitment and retention of staff in different disciplines, institutional and clinical philosophy, the past history of the institution or service, physical geography, and the professional and personal circumstances of its members at any one point. There may be the perception that an 'ideal' team make-up or membership exists, but the nature of health care and, in particular, forensic mental health care, is such that the team may require a considerable degree of flexibility, not only in terms of working practice, but also in its component parts at different times and in different circumstances. It should also be borne in mind that the actual day-to-day role of each member may need to change or adapt or even overlap with that of others in the team in certain circumstances.

Given the intense and, at some times, extraordinarily challenging nature of the work and the need to accommodate the important issue of patient involvement in decision-making, even in a secure or restricted environment or where there are clear legal constraints on some aspects of practice; the important issue of patient or user choice and involvement should not be allowed to become subservient to rigid institutionalised or establishment-based structures or practice. This may, therefore, for example, necessitate at times a change of personnel or of an individual working with a particular patient, actively withdrawing their involvement for a period. This inevitably leads to an alteration in the team's structure and membership, and to ways of working practice. Such a situation might involve clinicians working across more than one team and, indeed, this is commonplace in many areas of forensic practice simply as a matter of human resource allocation.

One might argue that the team should consist of a stable group of individuals who work closely together with a clearly defined client group and, for instance, responsibility for a geographical catchment area, or with a particular clinical remit, for instance, in intensive care, outpatient supervision or slow stream forensic rehabilitation, in order to optimise team functioning and interprofessional working and understanding of individual roles and capabilities. On the other hand, given the nature of the field, flexibility of approach may be equally important in particular situations. There may, for example, be occasions upon which patients are unwilling to be seen by one or another member of the team, but where an individual from another discipline, or with a different relationship with the person concerned by virtue of their professional role or particular personal attributes, might be readily able to continue to maintain an effective therapeutic involvement. Again, this would not involve the member of one professional group taking on the mantle of another, rather the involvement of one or perhaps more members of a team remaining involved with the patient where it is impracticable for others to do so. This would not, of course, be seen as a long-term solution but is just one example of what strength in depth a multidisciplinary team may draw upon in difficult circumstances should it and its members feel secure enough to work in this way.

Team members should, ideally, all bring an area of professional expertise and personal experience in the field with them to the team, and in many ways these will be unique to their profession and the individual concerned. Nevertheless, in a very broad sense, there may be areas in which there is considerable overlap in terms of professional responsibilities and areas of practice, personal attributes and styles of working, as well as the ability simply to do the job. That is not to say that, in general, individual team members should be expected to be multiskilled and able to take on one another's professional roles. On the contrary, the recognition and understanding, as well as open discussion of and agreement about professional boundaries and limitations, is an important part of providing a sound foundation to safe clinical practice. Open, frank and honest communication between all members of the multidisciplinary team, a sense of inclusion and, at least in terms of decision-making, involvement and empowerment, is a vital part of effective sharing of work and responsibility.

CLINICAL TEAMS, DEPARTMENTAL TEAMS, INTERAGENCY WORKING AND USER INVOLVEMENT

The multidisciplinary *clinical* team operates as a group of individuals within other structures and there are areas that overlap with alternative other forms of team domain. In the field of forensic mental health care in particular, multiagency working has been fostered and encouraged from relatively early on and, in the modern era, is very much the norm. Examples of health care professionals in the field combining their clinical team work and patient care with that of other, outside agencies, such as the probation service, the police, the courts and other criminal justice organisations, as well as education and social services in a broader sense, is a part of everyday practice. There are particular examples of this described in the literature (Wix, 1994; Geelan et al., 1998; Clark et al., 2002; Smith et al., 2003; Riordan et al., 2004) and later here. While, in the main, one would expect these interactions and working practices to enhance not only the care of the mentally disordered individual but also the practice of professionals concerned in the process, even with the best will in the world and the most favourable resources, as well as personal and corporate commitment, where those from widely different backgrounds come together to attempt to achieve what might, at first, be perceived as a common end, problems can arise in relation to divided loyalties, most particularly when health service workers and those with a primary role to do with the running of the criminal justice system are concerned. Difficulties may be evident in relation to the main agenda and requirements of each of the individuals and the groups or teams concerned, and in terms of the desired aims and outcomes of the process overall.

Particularly in the recent past in the UK in health care in general, there has been increasing emphasis, quite correctly, on the place of the user, consumer or patient, in determining their individual wishes in relation to their health needs, and also encouragement to become directly involved in shaping models of service delivery. Some would argue, therefore, that the patients themselves should be considered members of the clinical team. Whether this or some alternative form of approach is fully or even partially embraced, it is very clear now that there is no place in the care of those with mental illness and other mental health-related difficulties for complacency, professional exclusivity or an overwhelming and all-pervasive sense of paternalism. Given the nature of the field and the symptomatology of some forms of mental disorder, one must acknowledge the appropriate need for the use of compulsory measures at times but, although it seems trite to say, there should be appropriate involvement and consultation with patients at all stages of the process of care (Department of Health, 1999; Trivedi and Wykes, 2002).

INDIVIDUAL CLINICAL TEAM MEMBERS

This section is not intended to be in any way a definitive or comprehensive description of the training or working of individual clinical team members in a forensic mental health care setting. This could only be appropriately undertaken by individuals from each of those different disciplines that potentially make up the team as a whole. That in itself would be the subject of an entire volume. What follows, therefore, is an attempt to identify potential members of a forensic multidisciplinary clinical team and describe just some of the areas in which each of them may function as individual practitioners and members of a group, as well as certain ways in which, it might be argued, there can sometimes be some overlap, in terms of roles and responsibilities, some of which have already been alluded to.

Forensic mental health care nurses

Mental health nurses are the single largest professional group directly involved in the care of mentally disordered offenders and those who require similar services, and are also, therefore, arguably the most important. For inpatient settings at all levels of security, they have the most frequent and immediate and, in many cases, minute-to-minute clinical contact with patients throughout the entire day. Where forensic mental health patients are being followed up in the community, nurses play an equally important part in providing care and supervision to that undertaken by their professional counterparts in other disciplines (Kettles and Robinson, 2000). In hospitals, forensic nurses have a unique role in terms

of establishing and maintaining a close therapeutic relationship with patients and maintaining a foundation from which the other members of the clinical team can work. It has been shown that the quality of day-to-day relationships with nursing staff is, for patients detained in a secure environment and in contact with community forensic services, probably the most important single factor in user satisfaction with services (Riordan et al., 2004). Nursing staff dealing with forensic patients on an

inpatient unit are potentially able to establish an understanding of the patient's psychopathology, symptoms, and personal needs and wishes, in a way that no other discipline will, owing to the intensity and depth of involvement gained through constant day-to-day contact and interactions with service users, as well as clinical observation and assessment. On this basis, it could be argued that an experienced, senior, unit-based member of nursing staff is one of the most important and key members of any clinical team in forensic mental health care. This may not only be the case for a team dealing solely with inpatient management but can also be important in the context of community supervision of mentally disordered offenders by a team. The presence of a senior inpatient service-based nurse does not, nevertheless, preclude the involvement of a forensic community mental health nurse (FCMHN) on the team in addition.

One of the most important roles that can be fulfilled by a senior nurse in the team role is that of facilitating liaison between the team itself, with its multidisciplinary membership, unit-based nursing staff and the wider nursing establishment. This is vital in conveying specialist nursing issues to those from other disciplines and also in linking into those operational, practical and clinical matters, which primarily concern the nursing staff group working with the patient. In addition, there are likely at times to be nursing issues that may arise that it would not be appropriate for a member of any other professional group to deal with, such as those around professional standards of practice, for instance, in the same way as would apply to any of the other professional groups. The team's senior nurse will also obviously play a vital role in coordinating or undertaking assessments of patients for potential admission to inpatient care, and have an understanding of day-to-day service and clinical pressures at ward level that would not necessarily be available in the same way to other team members.

Forensic community mental health nurses

There is an argument, irrespective of whether the clinical team is involved in the care only of inpatients or whether it has responsibility for the supervision of outpatients also, for the inclusion of a specialist forensic community mental health nurse on the team in addition to the senior inpatient nurse member. Where the team is involved in the delivery of either outpatient services alone or carrying responsibility for inpatient beds as well as a parallel outpatient caseload, the presence of a forensic community psychiatric nurse as a member of the multidisciplinary team is a potentially important part of its successful functioning. The forensic community mental health nurse not only provides a link between the community and the team as a whole, but also may be in a position to advise on assessment for potential inpatient admission in the light of knowledge of community facilities and previous experience of involvement with service users following discharge and during the process of rehabilitation. The provision and administration of medication will only be a minor part of the FCMHN's role in the follow-up of mentally disordered offenders. The involvement of a number of people from a team, including the FCMHN, in the follow-up process is likely to be beneficial in terms of increased frequency of contact with the patient, the ability to assess and reassess their mental state, and the sharing of responsibility for supervision and management. Forensic community mental health nurses working in a particular geographical 'patch' are also likely to develop expertise in the knowledge of suitable community placements for discharged patients and get to know staff in other facilities, as well as those working within, for instance, the various criminal justice agencies, such as the police or court officers in a particular locality or area. There are, in addition, other ways in which FCMHNs may work in a liaison capacity within the forensic mental health field, for instance, through involvement with specialist bail hostel facilities, schemes for diversion at the point of arrest or at court, and in active liaison with local community mental health teams (Wix, 1994; Riordan et al., 2000).

Forensic mental health care social workers

Forensic social workers bring a wide range of skills and abilities to a multidisciplinary clinical team. They may fulfil the statutory role of social supervisor following conditional discharge of restricted hospital order patients but this may constitute only a very small part of their overall contribution. There is the potential, as with all other members of the team, to be involved in advising on the process of assessment, through admission to hospital, if this proves necessary for the patient concerned and then, most particularly perhaps, in moving on towards a placement beyond secure provision and into the community at large or to some form of an alternative health or social care facility. With expertise, knowledge and understanding of individual patients' clinical and social needs, and of the wide range of potential facilities for both inpatients and outpatients, the social worker may be the most important individual in identifying appropriate placements for patients once they are discharged from hospital. They may also be in a position to forge a particularly strong alliance with individual users and to take a more independent stance on clinical matters during the course of an inpatient stay, not being directly involved, for instance, in prescription or administration of medication, particularly if this is given against the patient's wishes.

The forensic mental health care social worker will often, if not almost always, take the lead role in contacting, and subsequently liaising with patients' relatives and other carers from the initial point of contact with the team right through to and following discharge from hospital. This relationship potentially provides a rich source of information during the course of the initial and subsequent assessment period, and equally importantly, a direct route of communication for patients with family members or friends, who may indeed already be close and supportive, but who might also have become distanced and alienated over time, as a result of difficulties in the past arising out of the patient's mental illness and its symptoms, or due to involvement as a victim or victims of the individual's offending behaviour.

Very often the forensic social worker will have a particular expertise and knowledge of mental health and other related, important, legislation, for instance, around incapacity, social care and finances. They may also possess approved social worker, or equivalent, status under the relevant Mental Health Act and, therefore, have a potentially important function in assessment or reassessment of patients who might need to be detained in hospital for whatever reason under civil procedures. In addition, they may fulfil the role of social supervisor for conditionally discharged restricted hospital order patients and, therefore, be required to provide a specific form of service to this particular user group as well as undertaking the statutory obligation of that role by producing the appropriate reports. As with their counterparts in general psychiatry services, they also have an important part to play in the provision of reports and oral evidence to the Mental Health Review Tribunal or its equivalent body elsewhere.

In terms of the process of assessment for possible admission to hospital, the forensic social worker will be able to address the issue of future placement even before an individual patient is brought in to hospital, for example, and, even at that relatively early stage, have an understanding of potential sources of information and contacts not available to other members of the team, for instance, through links with the wider social services network, education, probation and other agencies. Of course, an expertise in understanding benefits and sources of financial support for patients at all stages of contact with forensic services is an invaluable part of the forensic social worker's role as is liaison also with, for instance, the patient's legal representative. The social worker working in a forensic setting may also have a particular need for involvement at times in issues around child and vulnerable adult protection.

Clinical and forensic psychologists

The psychologist working in a forensic mental health team will have a degree-level qualification and then subsequent, prolonged and detailed, specialist postgraduate training and experience in the clinical and/or forensic fields. In terms of the team and its work, the psychologist, as with the other disciplines, may bring a different aspect and insight to the clinical and other tasks of the group depending on their particular area of interest. In a general sense, the team psychologist will have an ability to take an independent professional view of the team as a whole and its workings, and the clinical management of cases, and advise accordingly, as well as being a vitally important integrated part of the team with special skills in many areas, not least those of the use of structured assessment instruments for a range of different purposes, a sophisticated understanding of the variations in normal and abnormal human behaviour and, in particular, offending and its relationship with personality, individual histories and dynamic and developmental issues. The psychologist will also have experience and expertise in a range of psychological interventions and therapies not necessarily available to other team members. The psychologist is likely to bring an understanding and appreciation of the need for evidence-based practice and, in particular, research and its potential importance in the field of forensic mental health as a whole. In forensic settings, the psychologist is likely to have special skills in the assessment and management of risk, and may take a lead role in this aspect.

Forensic occupational therapists

Occupational therapists working in forensic settings and with forensic patients in the community bring their general professional skills in terms of detailed assessment and treatment of need and patients' individual abilities. In addition, they have a more specific understanding of the particular problems associated with patients who may have spent long periods in secure settings of one sort or another, including prisons and hospitals, who may also have a background of serious offending behaviour and who need particular forms of intervention and treatment that are peculiar to this patient group. Again, the occupational therapist working in a forensic mental health team will have an extremely important role to play in every stage of the process of a forensic patient's care, be that in the assessment process prior to admission to hospital, during the course of an inpatient's stay, in particular in relation to moves to lesser levels of secure care and then in the process of the patient's move into community living. Their training and expertise in particular forms of assessment is unique to the profession and in forensic rehabilitation, for instance, given appropriate resources, they may have as much, or more, day-to-day contact with patients as any of the other professional groups. Equally, they will have links with a range of agencies and other facilities and organisations in the community at large, such as day care centres, employment-related projects, voluntary bodies and statutory agencies, which places them in the position of being able to advise from a very wide knowledge base on individual patient need and how this might be matched with what is known to be available.

Pharmacists

A pharmacist as a member of a forensic mental health care clinical team, particularly one working in that specialist area alone, will develop a huge and detailed expertise in the pharmaceutical treatment of various forms of mental illness and disorders affecting forensic patients. These pharmacists are in a position to focus specifically on the use of medication and advise medical practitioners in their prescribing. They may have a role in compiling detailed drug histories, often in cases of resistant chronic illness where patients have received treatment for many years and, in addition, identify potential specific difficulties in terms of drug interactions or risks related to particular preparations, especially where the individual concerned has a complex general medical background or condition. Pharmacists may also have a role in identifying potential anomalies or problems where responsibility for prescribing for non-psychiatric conditions lies with, for instance, a visiting general practitioner (GP) providing services to an inpatient unit or in the community where the GP may not necessarily have an in-depth knowledge or experience of the use of a wide range of psychotropic medication.

One specific instance of a situation in which the pharmacist working in a forensic setting may be particularly well qualified to comment is in relation to the requirement under some current mental health legislation for any independent second opinion appointed doctor to consult with a non-nursing, non-medical team member who is involved with the patient's treatment in relation to the issue of assessment of consent to treatment with medication, where a patient is either incompetent or unwilling to give that consent. In these circumstances, the pharmacist is in a position to give an expert account of the treatment background and response over time, which will complement that of the medical and other professionals involved.

Forensic psychiatrists

The forensic psychiatrist is a medical practitioner with general professional training in psychiatry and then higher specialist training in the forensic mental health field. The psychiatrist has a background in the diagnosis of mental illness and other forms of mental disorder, and the assessment of normal and abnormal mental states and their treatment. In the forensic field, he or she will have a particular expertise in mental health legislation and its operation, the assessment, care and management of mentally disordered offenders, an understanding of criminal and civil legal processes and mental abnormality in the context of general medicine and physical well-being and ill health. The forensic psychiatrist will also almost certainly have had experience in working in different secure and non-secure, and other health care settings, as well as in prisons and the community. In addition, he or she will have been trained in matters relating to the provision of professional and expert advice to the courts. While forensic psychiatry is a relatively young subspecialty, it has expanded rapidly with increasing understanding of the relationship between mental disorder and offending behaviour, as well as with increasing concern over, to mention one area alone, the number of mentally ill people in prison. It is now established as a recognised branch of psychiatry in many parts of the world.

POTENTIAL CONFLICT AND TEAM LEADERSHIP

There are some ways in which difficulties may arise in teams in any context, let alone a very specialised area of health care. There may be potential or actual problems in relation to professional and personal status and roles, around issues of team aims and objectives, as well as leadership, effective management and interdisciplinary jealousies over working practice and boundaries. There may be reluctance on the part of some professionals to work with particular user or patient groups, where others would see this as clearly part of their core business. Many psychologists working in forensic settings, for example, would see the assessment, diagnosis and treatment of patients with personality disorder as a natural, and in some cases major part of their work, whereas some forensic psychiatrists might either not be so willing to be involved with this patient group or see their role more in relation to the diagnosis and treatment of mental illness, such as schizophrenia or major affective disorder alone.

As has already been indicated earlier, there may be variations in values and overall culture within different professional groups. For instance, clinical psychologists come very much from a background of evidence-based practice, and with an expectation of an ongoing involvement in investigation and research. Nurses, by contrast, have historically and traditionally had little grounding in research methodology or practice.

Team members will bring with them different skills as outlined and also, possibly, markedly different areas of specific interest. There are shared skills, such as correlation of information and history taking, as well as those which are central to the role of each individual discipline, for example, the use of drugs and therapeutics in psychiatry, or the application of specific instruments or tests in clinical or forensic psychology. There are also statutory requirements of some members of the team, which could lead either to professional envy on the one hand or, on the other, the possibility of a particular member of the team feeling overworked or pressured in one specific area. An example of this might be the need for the responsible medical officer and team social worker to produce reports to a specific deadline in relation to renewal of detention, applications to the Mental Health Review Tribunal and regular updates on restricted hospital order patients to the Home Office. This pressure may well affect the team as a whole in other areas, not least in relation to other mandatory requirements, such as Care Programme Approach review meetings and case conferences.

Conversely, there are huge strengths in working within a multidisciplinary group with a common purpose. Each individual brings a different area of expertise to bear on the same issue or issues, and patient care is, therefore, enhanced. There is the potential for sharing in decision-making and carrying responsibility and, given the right working atmosphere and sense of security within the team, the opportunity to put forward sometimes a very different, challenging or even opposing view in order to allow an exploration of all the possibilities. Griffin (1989) has described the multidisciplinary team as 'the integration of the separate perspectives, knowledge or skills of the healthcare professionals involved . . . without blurring of interdisciplinary boundaries . . . or loss of professional independence'. One might add that, in an ideal situation, team members should feel able to 'support one another in disagreement' (Thomas-Peter, personal communication).

TEAM LEADERSHIP

The word 'leader' is a noun that may be defined in terms of itself as a person who (or something which) leads or acts as the head, principal, main or chief individual or commander. However, the term 'leadership', to some extent, has come to imply a particular type of quality in an individual, in the political sphere as well as increasingly in that of business, management and health care delivery. It seems to suggest a combination of charisma, expertise and knowledge as well as power, coupled with the ability to make decisions and drive these forward, and a capacity to accept responsibility and carry others along, even if the direction in which the process is going is not that desired by all those involved. There is, therefore, potential confusion with issues around visionary attitudes, responsibility, accountability and authority, as well as delegation and status in relation to this issue and multidisciplinary team working. It might be argued that the word 'leadership' should be abandoned in favour of a detailed exploration, and then definitions of these other terms and their usage in order to avoid potential difficulties arising.

In the past, doctors have traditionally been a dominant force in the provision of health care to patients. Increasingly, this is no longer the case and, for a variety of reasons, the medical profession is coming under greater scrutiny, for instance, in the United Kingdom, in relation to performance-related audit, formal appraisal for all grades of doctor and consultant revalidation.

Even within multidisciplinary health care teams the prime responsibility of each individual member is to do with their relationship with the patient and the duty of care. In that sense, each individual team member carries their own professional accountability and no one person can be held responsible for the actions or omissions of another.

Case example 1

A 43-year-old man with a diagnosis of paranoid schizophrenia was being supervised by a forensic clinical team in the community under the terms of a restricted hospital order. He was seen regularly by his responsible medical officer and social supervisor, as well as the FCMHN. Over a period of some 3–4 months and with no other evident change in his mental state, he became convinced that the FCMHN was injecting him with poison rather than the appropriate depot medication and eventually refused to see her. It was agreed after discussion with the patient that he should attend the inpatient unit on a fortnightly basis where ward nurses who he knew well could administer his depot injection. After some months again it was suggested that an alternative FCMHN should visit him at home to give his medication and this was agreed. In a further 3 months the original FCMHN started to visit with her colleague on a fortnightly basis and eventually took over the role of monitoring the patient's progress and administering medication entirely with no reservations on the part of the patient or any concerns about the issue that had led to the original difficulties.

Case example 2

A 31-year-old man with a history of recurrent episodes of mania and extensive previous involvement with the criminal justice system was being followed up by a forensic clinical team as a voluntary outpatient. His main point of contact had always been through the senior social worker who he saw as being helpful in gaining assistance with finance, housing and potential employment. As a result of his concerns about continuing with mood-stabilising medication, he refused to continue to see the psychiatrist on the team. Despite this, he maintained his relationship and contact with his social worker and, as a result, when he showed the early warning signs of relapse of his illness, appropriate arrangements were quickly put in place for a mental health assessment, and the patient was admitted to hospital and had a brief admission during which he commenced medication again. His mental state rapidly improved and he could be discharged once more into the community and the relationship with his doctor and other members of the team was restored.

Case examples 1 and 2 illustrate the ways in which mental health care workers from the same or different professional groups may act in a variable capacity according to the immediate needs of the patient and their ongoing care. Case example 3 shows the value to strength in depth in terms of the wider institution and the larger forensic mental health care 'team' working within a particular service. This is reflected also in Case example 1 to some extent in that there were other members of the FCMHN department ready to pick up the care of that particular patient. In Case example 3, this ultimately involved a much broader change, made possible by the fact that there were other, similar, clinical teams working within the same set-up who were willing and able to consider taking over the patient's care, a solution which might not have been so readily available where only one or two forensic teams were working in parallel.

Case example 3

A woman of 32 years who had been an inpatient at a medium secure unit for two and a half years with unremitting severe psychotic symptoms made a formal complaint about her psychiatrist as he had not recommended her discharge from hospital at a Mental Health Review Tribunal. Several members of the clinical team discussed the situation with her at length, and both the Clinical Director of the unit and Complaints Manager, as well as the Service Director saw her at her own request. Despite the fact that all those concerned expressed the view that a change of RMO was unlikely to lead to any substantial difference in her care and management, she remained adamant in her wishes. She developed delusional beliefs about her consultant psychiatrist and refused to see him or allow any of the medical members of the team to assess her mental state at interview. It was agreed in negotiation with another clinical team that they would take over her care.

Case example 4

The clerk of a local magistrates' court referred a 26-year-old man for a psychiatric report. The probation officer allocated to produce a pre-sentence report thought that this man was known to psychiatric services, and had reported hearing voices telling him to harm others at the time of the offences he had committed had raised concerns. The magistrates and probation officer, as well as the man's legal representatives, thought it possible that he may be suffering from a mental illness and require treatment in hospital. This matter had been raised also by the arresting police officers and custody sergeant and, in addition, the police surgeon who had examined him some hours after his arrest. Despite this, there had been no sustained evidence of psychotic symptoms or mental illness during the course of the man's remand in custody and he had not been referred by the prison medical officer to the prison's visiting psychiatrist.

A detailed investigation of this individual's background and, in particular, his previous contact with psychiatric services, as well as clinical examination of his mental state following the request for the report, revealed repeated brief episodes of psychotic symptoms following the use of crack cocaine, which had consistently resolved within 10–12 hours on each previous occasion with no sustained evidence of mental illness. As the man himself did not see the need for any help with his illegal drug use and showed no motivation to change in this respect, no recommendation was put before the court in the psychiatric report and he was dealt with accordingly by due course of law.

This case description illustrates the way in which uncertainty and misinterpretation of this man's presentation might have led to an inappropriate outcome but where, ultimately, effective interagency liaison and consultation helped the process. Equally, there may be occasions on which, despite the best efforts of those involved, the opposite may occur, as illustrated in Case example 5 but in which, nevertheless, the outcome may also be the correct one. In considering these vignettes, however, it should be borne in mind how easy it can be for issues to become muddled and unclear. This can lead to confusion, a sense of frustration on the part of all those concerned and the inclination to approach similar situations and circumstance in the future with caution and scepticism about the abilities and motivation of others involved, despite all those concerned having acted in what they considered to be an appropriate manner and in keeping with conventional practices and expectations.

Case example 5

A community mental health nurse was called to a local police station to see a man who was causing concern to custody staff. He had reported feeling that life was no longer worth living. After thorough clinical review, it was clear that the man had been drinking heavily, but was now sober and had no enduring ideas or intentions of harm towards himself or others and, therefore, did not require or need immediate further input from psychiatric services, and could safely be given police bail.

On the way out of the custody suite, the FCMHN noticed on a wall chart record of detainees the name of a woman known to forensic mental health care services who had previously been given a diagnosis of personality disorder but also had a long history of intermittent episodes of severe psychosis. On further enquiry, it transpired that the police believed that the woman was not mentally unwell but making odd statements nevertheless. They had not intended to ask for a review of her mental state as, despite this, there were no concerns for her immediate safety, and she had frequently been in custody previously in similar circumstances and presenting in much the same way.

After further discussion, this woman was assessed by the FCMHN concerned, who found her to be floridly psychotic and distressed by a wide range of symptoms. An immediate mental health assessment was arranged and the patient was admitted to hospital under a civil compulsory order.

A similar issue to that pertaining to the potential difficulties of multiagency working arises in relation to those from the different mental health care groups in multidisciplinary clinical teams. They may each be a member, not only of that group, but also of a department consisting of clinicians all from the same professional background, or another subgroup or, for instance, committee, whose structure, objectives and desired ends might be quite different from that of the clinical team itself.

Matters may be discussed, or decisions considered or taken within the clinical team and, for example, a departmental team meeting or within a general management orientated setting, which are potentially contradictory or seemingly fundamentally opposed to one another. In this situation, team members may find themselves in a difficult position or feel at risk of compromising their relationship with members of their own professional group and also those with whom they are most closely concerned in providing day-to-day patient care in the multidisciplinary team.

Case example 6

A 35-year-old man with chronic schizophrenia was placed in a rehabilitation unit of a medium-secure facility. Following extensive discussion and review, what seemed an appropriate future community placement was identified by the team social worker. Visits were arranged as a part of the patient's rehabilitation programme and these were commenced. In the mean time, the purchasing authority had decided to open a refurbished community unit of its own and withdrew support for the patient's move to the previously identified residential facility. The situation was only resolved, initially with the involvement of the patient's solicitor, and then by an extensive process of consultation, whereby an understanding was reached that the earlier placement was far more suited to the needs of the particular individual concerned than that which had subsequently been proposed, and would, therefore, be less likely to break down, or to lead to a relapse of the patient's mental illness, and an undesirable and unnecessarily prolonged period in hospital again.

In these circumstances, the forensic mental health care team social worker had been placed in a difficult position, having identified a suitable community facility that had been discussed within clinical team meetings and agreed as being appropriate, only then to discover later, initially through a briefing at a departmental meeting, that the particular purchaser concerned had taken a blanket decision to agree only to move patients requiring forensic rehabilitation into one particular unit, thus compromising the clinical decision made earlier.

CLINICAL TEAM MEETINGS

Just as there is no set rigid requirement in terms of multidisciplinary team membership in forensic mental health care work, so there is no set format or configuration for multidisciplinary clinical team meetings. The timing, structure and process of these will vary depending, again, upon the setting, the user group, and team membership and working practices. There has been an unwritten tradition, within hospital medical practice, of the weekly ward round or its equivalent. In the various branches of physical medicine and surgery, this has taken the form of medical staff and ward nurses moving from one bed to the next around the unit discussing patients' care, talking to them, examining them, and ordering investigations or planning the next stage of treatment. This has tended to be a part of the accepted routine. Sometimes, these formal reviews have been supplemented by other rounds undertaken by junior medical staff, and any additional involvement has been on an as-required or needs-based footing.

In psychiatry, this approach has evolved more towards the model of a regular, often again weekly, meeting where those involved in the patients' care gather to discuss progress and developments in each case, with the individual themselves then invited to attend and discuss the various recommendations and potential outcomes. The length of time spent in this way, the day of the week, and whether morning or afternoon or both, those attending and the format of these meetings can vary widely, and have essentially been arbitrary and may depend to some extent at least on logistics and the personal preferences of those involved. There may also, of course, be institutional considerations that play a part, for instance, where a unit or units have patients who are involved with a number of different teams, which might, therefore, hold their clinical review meetings at different times.

In any branch of health care, the process of assessment and updating of treatment and management plans is a continuous one and, in hospital medicine, is a continuous part of day-to-day practice. Nevertheless, the formal meeting fulfils not only the purpose of reviewing patients' treatment but also provides a regular point of contact with one another for those working in the same team. This can be as important a function of the regular team meeting as is the opportunity to review the team's clinical work and involvement with individual patients. In mental health care and, in particular, forensic mental health care settings, where many service users will be subject to the requirements of the Care Programme Approach, this format also provides a structure within which to set the necessary regular review process that is required. A regular team meeting allows not only for the conduct of necessary clinical and related business, but informal discussion of other direct patient care-related matters, institutional and management issues affecting the team, problems in any particular areas and the sharing of concerns or in decision-making that do not relate specifically to the normal, or scheduled, content of the meeting. It provides a focus for team members to meet in what is hopefully, for most of those involved, protected time, and a forum for discussion, exchange of ideas, obtaining the views of those who might bring a different perspective to particular issues and a source of mutual support. It may, in fact, reduce the need for more frequent, informal, contact at other times in that each team member will know that they will see the others at a particular point in the week and may, therefore, be able to hold on to issues for discussion until then.

There are a variety of possible different formats to clinical team meetings in forensic mental health care and the discussion here is not intended to be exhaustive. Rather, the aim is to suggest some ways in which those involved might consider conducting and organising clinical team meetings.

The frequency of meetings is inevitably arbitrary. For the majority of teams, this will be on a weekly basis. The timing of the meeting will be a matter for the team members themselves to decide and agree upon. There may be particular advantages or disadvantages to holding meetings on certain days of the week or in the morning or afternoon, which again are for the team and its members to reach a consensus about. Depending upon the volume of work and the necessary ground to be covered on each occasion, the length of the meeting may vary considerably. Some teams may only meet for an hour or two, whereas others may spend a full working day, or possibly more, on the multidisciplinary team business.

There will be variation in the order of discussion or the actual content of the clinical team meeting. There may be circumstances in which all the team's work is reviewed on each and every occasion, and others where this might not be the case. For instance, it may be that there is a set format or agenda organised and ordered before the meeting commences, with certain standing and other variable items. Patient care and clinical management may be reviewed at different intervals, for instance, weekly or fortnightly, depending on their progress and placement or, possibly in other circumstances, on a less frequent but more in-depth basis. The team may wish to include discussion of new referrals to team members at some point during the course of the meeting, any specific difficulties with areas of clinical work that are not due to be formally reviewed and then undertake the more formalised business of clinical review. Some teams will have a nominated chairperson or persons. Others might be more 'naturalistic', with a less structured approach to presentation and discussion. Some teams may rotate the role and responsibilities of coordinating and running the meeting between its members on a regular basis, allowing each to take a lead at different points in time and others to move to a position of less direct involvement in the actual mechanics of the process itself.

There may be a separate period of time set aside for the discussion of new referrals and the progress of ongoing assessments. In addition, the team may choose to combine with its regular team meeting, formal case conference reviews linked to clinical requirements and the Care Programme Approach. If the team is managing both inpatients and outpatients, there will have to be a consideration of when and where community patients are reviewed by the team as a whole, and it may be that this forms part of the regular multidisciplinary team meeting, is an entirely separate undertaking, or that it replaces one of the regular weekly meetings, for instance, as part of a monthly cycle.

The way in which the team conducts itself and the team meetings take place will be very much a function of the decisions made by its members about how and when they wish to have their meeting, how the business will be transacted, and what it will consist of and how long it will take. Inevitably, as with the overall character of the team itself, its meetings and their tone and character will depend very much on the make-up of the team and the personalities of those involved, and their interpersonal skills and interactions. Its success depends to a great extent on the ability of all those involved to recognise the expertise, abilities and potential contribution of others to the work of the team as a whole, and the need to remain focused but work together towards an agreed goal. This end may be achieved in a variety of different ways but will, nevertheless, remain the ultimate aim of the team's members together. Teams that operate in a hierarchical fashion may not be so effective or contented as those where the principle of a 'flattened democracy' is more predominant. This depends, to a great extent, on how secure each member of the team feels in the company of the others and how able they feel to put forward their views no matter how seemingly obvious or potentially controversial. In the end, the team needs to keep as its central focus the best interests of its patient group and work through individual differences to maintain that (Burrow, 1999).

References

Burrow S (1999) The forensic multidisciplinary care team. In Tarbuck P, Topping-Morris B and Burnard P (eds) Forensic mental health nursing: policy, strategy and implementation. London: Whurr Publishers

Clark T, Kenney-Herbert J P, Baker J and Humphreys M S (2002) Psychiatric probation officers: failed provision or future panacea? Medicine, Science and the Law 42: 58–63

Department of Health (1999) Patient and public involvement in the new NHS. London: HMSO

Geelan S, Griffin N and Briscoe J (1998) A profile of the residents at Elliott House: the first bail and probation hostel for mentally disordered offenders. Health Trends 30: 101–105

Griffin N (1989) Multi professional care in forensic psychiatry. Psychiatric Bulletin 13: 613–615

Kettles A and Robinson D (2000) Overview and contemporary issues in the role of the forensic nurse in the UK. In: Kettles A and Robinson D (eds) Forensic nursing and multidisciplinary care of the mentally disordered offender. London: Jessica Kingsley Publishers

Riordan S, Wix S, Kenney-Herberth J and humphreys M (2000) Diversion at the point of arrest: A description of Mentally disordered individuals early contact with the police in Birmingham. Journal of Forensic Psychiatry 3: 683–690

Riordan S, Lyons K and Humphreys M S (2004) Pathways to medium secure care in Birmingham and patient perceptions. Research report. Birmingham: NHS West Midlands Regional Health Authority

Smith S S, Baxter V J and Humphreys M S (2003) Psychiatric treatment in prison: a missed opportunity? Medicine Science and the Law 43: 122–126

Trivedi P and Wykes T (2002) From passive subjects to equal partners. British Journal of Psychiatry 181: 468–472

Wix S (1994) Keeping on the straight and narrow: diversion of mentally disordered offenders at the point of arrest. Psychiatric Care 1: 102–104

Chapter 4

Specific joint working I

Chapter 4A
The role of the manager

Kate Lyons

> To manage is to forecast and plan, to organize, to command, to co-ordinate and to control.
>
> (Henri Fayol, 1916)

INTRODUCTION

Since the development of the National Health Service (NHS) in 1948, the role of the manager has been evolving and changing. Initially, the term used for this role was 'administrator' but, over time, it has been recognised that 'manager' more adequately reflects the duties and responsibilities of those concerned. Regrettably, the attitudes of both the public and, also to an extent, clinicians towards management in the NHS have often been somewhat negative as to its place and relevance. In an organisation as complex as modern-day United Kingdom health services, the manager is, nevertheless, an essential component of the overall team who can support and inform the process of clinical activity, allowing health care professionals to focus on patient-related matters. Working in cooperation with clinicians, the properly trained, experienced manager is able to provide many of the key planning and organisational skills to ensure continuous quality improvement and service development in health care settings.

THE ROLE OF THE MANAGER

One might reasonably ask 'Where and how does the manager fit in a multidisciplinary team environment in the NHS?' The multidisciplinary team may operate at different levels, for instance, the localised clinical team managing a specific caseload, the multidisciplinary management team taking a lead responsibility for managing a service area or directorate, or the multidisciplinary executive team managing an entire organisation. The manager has a role to play in each of these, which may be fixed over time or vary according to circumstances. Generally, the 'local' multidisciplinary clinical team managing its own caseload will have more limited, although no less important at times, involvement from a manager on a day-to-day basis as they take forward individual patient care. The role of the manager at directorate level will be far more influential in ensuring services as a whole are managed efficiently and effectively, and developed in line with corporate objectives and local and national service strategy. At executive organisational level, the role of the manager will vary depending on their own degree of seniority, for example, the directorate manager may provide a 'bridge' between the executive and operational levels, whilst the manager as part of a multidisciplinary executive team is likely to have a much more focused strategic role in leading the organisation.

THE THEORY OF THE MANAGER'S ROLE

When looking at the specific role of the manager in the context of the multidisciplinary health care team, even if for reasons of practicality in a limited way, it is essential to review some of the theory of management as a whole. The variety of interpretations of the managerial role perhaps reflects the wide-ranging nature of the potential tasks to be undertaken.

Henry Mintzberg (1973) developed a list of activities that he saw as commonly part of the role, particularly, of senior managers. He divided these into three main areas: interpersonal, informational and decisional. While this model may be helpful, it should be recognised that many of the areas described are not mutually exclusive and that there is considerable overlap.

Urwick (1975) has similarly identified ten principles that underpin the management role. Brech (1975) defined management as: 'A social process entailing responsibility for the effective and economical planning and regulation of the operations of an enterprise, in fulfilment of given purposes or tasks. . . .' He identified management as having four main elements, these being:

- planning
- control
- coordination
- motivation.

There are, of course, other theories. The reader is directed for a review to Drucker (1968) who considers the issue of management thinking in 'The practice of management'.

The areas outlined by both Mintzberg and Brech can be identified in many NHS managerial roles at many different levels within the organisation. In some circumstances, certain aspects will be more prominent than others, and reflect the nature of the management role and the specific situation varying with the level of seniority at which the individual or individuals concerned are operating. The higher in the organisation one looks, the more likely it is that all ten aspects identified by Mintzberg will be more clearly evident. An important feature to note about management in this context also is that, within a range of different circumstances and situations, the manager will deliberately act in different roles, for example, facilitator, partner, negotiator, decision-maker or leader in order to identify and then achieve certain objectives.

THE NHS CONTEXT

There have been a number of management reviews in the NHS over the last 25 years and subsequent role and structural redefinition. One of the key changes came in 1983 following the Griffiths Report (Department of Health, 1983), which reviewed 'effective use and management of manpower and related resources in the health service'. This document reinforced the concept of 'general management' by trying to define the role and responsibilities of the manager in the context of UK health care services as a whole. Most recently, 'Managing for excellence in the NHS' (Department of Health, 2002a) was published along with the 'Code of conduct for NHS managers' (Department of Health, 2002b). This was in response to the significant modernisation agenda set out in the NHS Plan and National Service Frameworks. At its launch, Sir Nigel Crisp, NHS Chief Executive at the time, identified that 'Modernisation of the NHS and the delivery of the NHS Plan constitute not only the biggest healthcare project in the world, they add up to the toughest management task as well'.

The 'Code of conduct for NHS managers' sets out core standards that underpin the role of the NHS manager. 'Managing for excellence in the NHS' outlines management reform and proposes a changing culture to ensure modernisation of the NHS and delivery of the NHS Plan.

The key tasks facing the managers of the future at that time were identified as being to work even more closely with clinicians in managing services, to focus more on working with patients, local communities and staff, and to learn new skills to implement changes. Underpinning the future of management development, the implementation of the Code of Conduct placed an expectation on managers in all health care Trusts to incorporate the code into chief executive and directors, contracts as well as any other senior managers for whom it was considered applicable. Each individual manager was expected to sign up to the following statement. 'As an NHS manager, I will observe the following principles:

- make the care and safety of patients my first concern and act to protect them from risk;
- respect the public, patients, relatives, carers, NHS staff and partners in other agencies;
- be honest and act with integrity;
- accept responsibility for my own work and the proper performance of the people I manage;

- show my commitment to working as a team member by working with all my colleagues in the NHS and the wider community;
- take responsibility for my own learning and development.'

This firmly enforced the need for managers to work closely alongside clinicians from all disciplines.

Some of the skills required to deliver the modernisation of the NHS through 'managing for excellence' are recognised to be:

- managing people;
- changing behaviour and influencing culture;
- managing information;
- effective communication;
- resource management;
- strategic planning;
- leadership.

The next section explores further the role of the manager working in a multidisciplinary environment taking into consideration the principles outlined above and with particular reference to forensic mental health care.

WHERE DOES THE MANAGER FIT?

To be most effective and to be able to continue to work within the principles described previously, it is essential that the health services manager is not isolated from clinical activity and behaves, and is seen by others, both externally and from within the organisation, as a member of the multidisciplinary team at all levels. There will undoubtedly be tensions as the wider remit of manager to take forward the corporate agenda, including its financial aspects, may at times be seen to be, or perceived as being, at odds to some extent at least, with clinical views. Mullins (1989), however, has stated that 'management is not a separate, discrete function'. An organisation cannot have a department of management in the same way as a department for other functions. Management is seen best, therefore, as a process common to all other functions carried out within the organisation. Management is essentially an integrating activity.'

Using examples of day-to-day working in a specialist forensic mental health care service will illustrate how the manager's role integrates and may become part of the clinical work of the institution and wider service, whilst still maintaining the general management overview to ensure, for instance, that financial stability is retained and performance targets are achieved.

SETTING THE SERVICE CONTEXT

In order to understand some of the processes of specialist health care management working, it is important to appreciate the service overall in order to set the context. A forensic service will almost always be part of a larger mental health organisation concerned with the provision of general, as well as other specialist forms of mental health care. Forensic mental health services will often have multidisciplinary management teams who together are responsible for the overall strategic direction and planning of the service. This may include the service director and operational manager, along with clinical heads of department and others, such as representatives from human resources or estates and facilities. This model is outlined in Figure 4.1.

SOME PRACTICAL EXAMPLES

This section, by reference to specific examples of joint working, describes the role of the manager at the three levels identified earlier, namely working with the individual clinical team, working within the directorate team and working within the wider organisation.

Working with the individual clinical team

As a manager, a key aspect of the role in, for instance, the directorate setting within the wider Trust, may be to assist and enable the resolution of potential or actual problems when there are, for instance, blocks in the system. This can be exemplified in a range of day-to-day circumstances, such as supporting a clinical team with a complex or delayed discharge, which requires negotiation over appropriate placement support or funding. It can also be necessary and appropriate for the manager to, as it were, remove the matter of finances from the equation, allowing clinicians to make decisions based on patient needs alone.

If one considers the example of discharge of patients from in-patient secure psychiatric services, then the role played by the manager in this aspect of day-to-day practice clearly includes supporting clinicians in making contact with the relevant parties, identifying the funding authority, ensuring necessary information is supplied to all parties and participation in meetings to discuss the appropriate resolution to a case as well as quite often taking on something of a lead role in the negotiations in some instances. This type of work is an essential part of the management role when the situation arises, where movement is halted and putting forward the case for change from a non-clinical perspective in the longer term can ensure both the improvement of the patient's experience and care, and enable the clinical team to achieve the desired objectives and outcome.

Figure 4.1 The multidisciplinary management team.

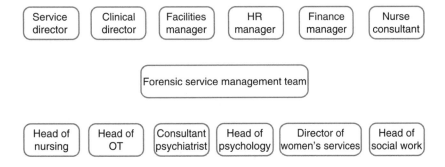

Case example 1

The clinical team planned to discharge the patient to an independent residential establishment and needed appropriate funding. After some weeks of correspondence and informal visits to the proposed placement by the patient, the team was unable to resolve the matter and referred to the service manager for assistance.

The role of the manager in this case was twofold. Firstly, to identify the block to the process, namely, that the key relevant individual in the process was no longer in post and that the central placement budget was overspent, so that no one else wished to make the decision, and then to find a solution by negotiation and liaison with all the other relevant parties.

As a manager, it is part and parcel of the job to understand the relevant bureaucracy and identify solutions. This case was resolved by returning to the funding authority and making plain not only the positive patient benefits that were to come from the move, but also the fact that the proposed accommodation would be far less expensive in the longer term.

Case example 2

A patient required urgent transfer from medium to high security for treatment but this did not seem possible in the timescale required. The impact of the patient remaining inappropriately placed was widespread and not in the interests of the individual concerned. The manager supported the clinical team by introducing an additional route into the transfer discussions, engaging the wider organisation for senior support and liaising with commissioners to obtain additional impetus. As the manager, making some of the chasing calls and supporting staff with regular progress reports was essential to maintain the day-to-day working environment in which the patient was placed until the transfer was made.

Working within the directorate management team

This is a significant role for many managers who bridge the operational and strategic elements of the organisation and its working practice. There are a number of examples of the ways in which the role of the manager may contribute in these areas.

Example 1—Managing the work

Referring back at the diagram of the multidisciplinary management team (Figure 4.1), it is possible to see the variety and range of disciplines within the overarching management structure. Each has a role both in providing a 'management view' and a 'professional view' to the team to allow services to be developed and to make decisions about the day-to-day running of the organisation. The manager working within the wider environment also has a multifaceted role, which includes facilitating debate and discussion, ensuring agreement or consensus can be achieved, drawing plans together, and often taking forward and supporting action and monitoring progress. This can include managing tensions between various professional groups and/or individuals depending on the organisational culture.

A specific example of this would be the introduction of performance indicators and the manager's role in ensuring delivery. Such a role would include gaining service ownership of targets, influencing the culture, facilitating clear communication and managing information. It also encompasses measuring performance and being able to agree priorities for action. Given some of the negativity that currently surrounds national targets in many public sector services, gaining support for, and being clear about the advantages of taking forward performance-related matters, is a key role of the NHS manager. If one considers many of the definitions of management described, then this aspect of coordinating and working through a multidisciplinary management team encompasses most, if not all of them.

Example 2– Negotiating funding and priorities

It is essential to allow clinicians to focus on providing patient care and services. However, it is also vital for them to influence service delivery and direction. With close working, the manager within the team is able to take forward much of this process. Health care provision is subject to regular review and renegotiation between commissioners and providers of services. The gathering and synthesis of information, and its use in identifying needs and promoting strengths together with clinical colleagues, is undoubtedly a key domain for the manager.

Discussion will always be required to prioritise the needs of the service and its development, and to identify pressures and areas for change to be discussed with commissioners. This will generally take place in a range of fora to ensure clinical ownership and is clearly within the spirit of the 'Managing for excellence in the NHS' framework of working closely with clinicians. The management role in these circumstances is in bringing together the main themes by leading much of the discussion, providing an overview of the financial and organisational context, ensuring prioritisation of demand and coordinating the interactions with commissioners. Currently, in the UK, the annual service, workforce and financial framework discussions require the manager to work with clinicians to develop proposals for consideration and to oversee the internal and external relationships. This function also requires the manager to understand and reflect local and national targets and strategies in discussions, and in taking developments forward, to ensure service direction and change is in line with these. If one considers Mintzberg's thinking on management tasks, this undoubtedly encompasses those of negotiator and liaison worker.

Example 3–Leading service development and change

When considering service development or change, obtaining consensus on the way forward with a large clinical group can be a challenging and, at times, seemingly insurmountable task. However, given disagreement or simple lack of common ground on issues, it may be necessary for the manager to arbitrate, to influence or to make a decision. Providing this is done in the context of listening to views, participation in debate and with due respect for the differing perspectives of others, this managerial role can be key to achieving an end result.

The manager will need to be able to take on the role of leadership within a multidisciplinary team. Huczynski and Buchanan (1991) have suggested that 'A manager can be regarded as someone who by definition is assigned a position of leadership in an organization'. However, they also assert that this does not mean all managers can be considered to be leaders. The skill of the leader in these circumstances is to allow for development of ideas to occur, to listen to the views of others and to support members of the team, whilst not be stifled or paralysed by a desire to consult and please everyone. This can be exemplified by an issue such as providing a business case in relation to change in facilities and services. In dealing with a potentially contentious issue, such as, for instance, the introduction of facilities to allow for seclusion of patients in a secure psychiatric or other mental health care facility where these have not previously been available, the manager needs to use a range of techniques to ensure that the move forward to a decision, whatever that decision might be, can occur. Recognising the issue, understanding barriers and articulating the advantages and disadvantages of each side of the discussion is an essential role that the manager can fulfil. Undertaking an options appraisal to determine possible solutions is also an essential component. One-to-one discussion, single-discipline discussions to gain an understanding of certain professional perspectives and multidisciplinary discussion to allow cross-boundary agreement, as well as the challenging of views, are all techniques that might be used. The skills of communication, changing behaviour and listening are all essential components of the management role in such circumstances.

Example 4—Managing the day-to-day finances

The manager must support clinicians to understand the overall strategic and financial context in which the service operates but not burden individual clinicians or attempt to influence clinical work for financial ends. It is in this environment that the main tension between clinicians and managers may come to the fore.

Interestingly, the Code of Conduct principle for managers that makes 'the care and safety of patients my first concern' is also a potential source of conflict within the management role, as a demanding financial agenda may be at risk of becoming too influential in some decision-making. How does the manager balance the requirement to secure income, for instance, against clinical need and the service pressure being so great that the admission of disturbed patients might compromise the safety, both of that individual and staff? This can be answered in part by the manager in some way ensuring ownership by the overall multidisciplinary management team of the financial framework and budgetary constraints that may exist in order to ensure those delegated responsibility for decision-making, and then service delivery, work within those. In supporting this, the manager should take the lead in financial control and resource allocation on a day-to-day basis. This includes close budgetary monitoring, including taking responsibility for the delivery of any savings targets or cost improvement programmes.

Example 5—Management involvement at all levels

The manager must provide active leadership and coordination for the service as a whole. From experience, it is poor practice for an NHS manager to remain isolated and away from other members of the team be they clinical, administrative or managerial workers. The 'team' should be considered a broad group and encompass those involved in all aspects of the service in order to ensure that staff feel valued in their contribution. The manager should ensure the involvement of all those employed in the service by utilising a range of techniques, including holding two-way briefing or workshops on strategy, for instance, as well as being available for one-to-one discussion and feedback with the staff and maintaining an approachable manner.

Good understanding of the services provided by specialist forensic mental health care units, their needs, those of patients, and staff morale and development come from some basic actions. It is imperative for a manager to be seen, that is, to be evident on a day-to-day basis, to be supportive, to be capable of taking action and, perhaps above all, to be involved. Many managers talk about 'walking the shop floor', which is an essential component to understanding staff issues, as well as dealing with matters that could become contentious if not addressed early and generally listening to staff views on a range of topics. Without this, the manager's credibility is affected, and he or she risks becoming isolated from those with whom they must maintain close contact to ensure the provision of effective, acceptable and safe services to patients. They also risk losing support and openness to ideas and change.

Working within the wider organisation

The performance of any specific service area is key to the overall success of an organisation in meeting its corporate objectives. As a manager within a clinical setting, there is a significant element of the role, which is about working between corporate and directorate levels, and actively working with the multidisciplinary team. Examples of this include reflecting the overall organisational objectives at directorate level, often through the management team or joint working with specific professional groups, as well as meeting the performance management targets of the organisation. The manager needs to have an understanding of the organisation as a whole to ensure the directorate is part of the overall body, and not isolated and working to a different agenda.

The role of the manager in this area, then, is undoubtedly to provide a bridge between the corporate team to allow them to be linked to the service, and also to ensure that issues are raised with a wider audience where appropriate. The manager from any given service area needs to know which issues require discussion at which level. Examples of this within a secure service might be, for instance, highlighting pressures of patient dependency impacting on the level of risk being managed with the service overall. It could also include obtaining support for decisions, such as reducing bed numbers in an inpatient setting to reduce risk, but equally taking into consideration the impact this might have on, for example, both patients, clinicians elsewhere, referring agencies and the organisation's financial position.

A further example of working with the wider organisation is in managing public relations issues and publicity. This may be particularly important in forensic mental health services, where high-profile individuals may be placed or which for other reasons may be of particular interest or concern to the wider community. The manager may act in a variety of ways in this respect, supporting and advising clinical colleagues, liaising with press relations officers or dealing with enquiries.

Given that forensic services can present a high risk, clinically, financially and publicly, the role of the manager is essential in maintaining local stability in service, whilst involving the wider organisation as required. Such management activities can be seen as a balancing act between operating within the organisation structures and knowing when to engage others.

SUMMARY

Being an NHS manager in a multidisciplinary environment can be extremely rewarding, but is not without its challenges, frustrations, and tensions. The NHS manager can at times feel undervalued by the public, by clinicians and by politicians alike, particularly when funding-related issues are high on the agenda and resources are said to be 'wasted' on non-clinical time. Nevertheless, the role is now an essential component of the organization, bringing a set of skills required to support delivery of effective and efficient services in the current NHS environment.

References

Department of Health (1983) The Griffiths Report. London: HMSO

Department of Health (2002a) Managing for excellence in the NHS. London: HMSO

Department of Health (2002b) Code of conduct for NHS managers. London: HMSO

Drucker P F (1968) The practice of management. London: Heinemann

Fayol H (1916) General and industrial management. London: Pitman. [Quoted from Cole G A (1988) Management theory and practice, 2nd edn. London: DP Publications]

Huczynski A and Buchanan D (1991) Organisational behaviour, 2nd edn. Engelwood Cliffs, NJ: Prentice Hall

Mintzberg H (1973) The nature of managerial work. London: Harper and Row

Mullins L (1989) Management and organisational behaviour, 2nd edn. London: Pitman

Urwick L F (1975) Elements of administration. In: Brech E F L (ed.) Principles and practice of management, 3rd edn. London: Longman

Suggested reading

Department of Health (2000) The NHS Plan: a plan for investment, a plan for reform. London: HMSO

Chapter 4B
The place of a legal representative or advocate working for their client

Philip J. Kenny

INTRODUCTION

The need for joint working between members of a patient's clinical team, public protection bodies and purchasers is readily apparent. The role of the patient's legal representative or advocate in working with the multidisciplinary team is less so. In a forensic setting, a clinical team's first point of contact with a prospective patient's legal team and quite possibly their advocate will often, although not always, be during the course of criminal proceedings. Once the court has dealt with the patient, a different legal team, quite possibly a different legal firm, will often become involved.

OVERVIEW OF THE ROLE

Many mental health legal representatives and advocates act on behalf of their client throughout, from the early days of their admission to the point of discharge and beyond. The discharge process itself will undoubtedly be a major concern for many patients, in particular, their right to apply to a Mental Health Review Tribunal. The patient's prospects of achieving a satisfactory outcome at a tribunal hearing will often depend upon the quality of the aftercare package to be put in place, and complex issues, such as the availability and suitability of accommodation, funding and follow-up arrangements. Individual patients' clinical teams may meet frequently to discuss the individual's progress and a wider range of agencies and their representatives come together at Care Programme Approach (CPA) review meetings. Patient involvement in such meetings may vary considerably and it is here, as well as at other important times, that the patient's legal representative may have a particularly important part to play. During the course of their detention, it is not uncommon for patients to have concerns with regard to specific aspects of their treatment, or to wish to pursue informal or formal complaints arising from a wide range of issues. Significant numbers of forensic patients are managed in the community, under the terms of a conditional discharge granted by the Home Office or by the Mental Health Review Tribunal (MHRT) and most will, in due course, wish to seek absolute discharge. The quality of communication between patients, their carers and concerned others, can significantly affect the quality of outcome for the patient and in turn for society as a whole.

Over the years, in both forensic and non-forensic settings, in hospital and in the community, many psychiatric patients, their carers and others involved in their lives, have consistently voiced their concern, at what they perceive to be a lack of effective communication on the part of those responsible for patient care. All of these concerns cannot satisfactorily be explained as being either illness related or resulting from a misunderstanding of how the process, as a whole, might work. Some of the causes are system failure and some the result of the inevitable fact that not all competent professionals are necessarily good communicators. In turn, the communication by or with individual legal representatives or advocates in such circumstances will in part depend upon the personal qualities of the individual, their ability to instil confidence in their client and to relate to the diverse personalities and clinical disciplines that make up a multidisciplinary team. Closer cooperation between a patient's clinical team and his or her legal adviser or advocate can give rise not only to improved communication, but also to a greater sense of involvement and resulting confidence in their care on the part of the patient. Whilst in some circumstances a legal representative or advocate may be required, either by their client's instructions or the particular circumstances of an individual matter, to adopt an adversarial approach, courts and tribunals alike are increasingly encouraging all parties to potential legal disputes, to adopt non-adversarial resolution policies and procedures. Whilst some clinical teams and their members, either as individuals or collectively, might view the involvement of legal representatives or advocates in the process of consultation and decision-making around clinical care as a potential means to seek ammunition for adversarial challenge, there is now an increasing and very welcome trend towards greater openness, with both patients and their legal advisers.

Each patient is an individual whose needs, wishes and abilities will change from time to time. Many will perceive themselves as being out of their depth, in dealing with what they may see as the power of the clinical team, their apparent inability to influence their present and future treatment, the complexity of the legal process and the absence of anyone who they perceive to be on their side. From this position of apparent disempowerment, some will seek to retain a very close control over the relationship between the clinical team and their legal representative or advocate. Some will insist that the relationship is conducted on an adversarial basis.

The majority choose neither of these courses and are relieved to be able to pass over some of what they see as the burden of dealing with the system and parts of it and the process, particularly of compulsory care and treatment, to a person in whom they can have confidence.

Some patients will benefit from the services of an advocate, some the services of a legal representative, and some may need or wish for both. The clinical team may, as a result, need to manage relationships with both an advocate and a legal representative, with the legal representative, in some instances, receiving their instructions through the patient's advocate.

For many individuals, the mere presence of someone 'on their side' at a meeting or with them on the ward will often enable patients to express their own views, without recourse to the services of the representative. This will in turn often facilitate the informal resolution of concerns, apparent problems, potential grievances and complaints, without recourse to more formal procedures.

Case example 1

P had been in conditions of medium security for about 3 years. He had concerns in relation to what he perceived to be the shortcomings of several members of his clinical team, which he believed were delaying his progress towards conditional discharge. P was of the opinion that his clinical team never listened to him when he was attempting to express his point of view, would not listen to his current concerns and would hold any representations he made against them as further evidence of mental illness. He thought the only way forward for him was to make a formal complaint to the Clinical Director. P was persuaded to allow his solicitor to arrange a review meeting with all of his clinical team present at which he could put forward his concerns supported by his legal representative. At the subsequent meeting, P put forward his concerns, his clinical team took on board his sense of frustration and their explanation of some of the matters helped P to understand the reason for some of the delays. The clinical team accepted that some of the delays could have been avoided and agreed ways of moving outstanding matters forward. P said later that the outcome of the meeting had not been as he had expected. He felt that the meeting had resulted in real progress and that it had been preferable to deal with the matter in this way rather than through use of the formal complaints procedure.

Ethnic minority patients are often significantly disadvantaged where they do not speak or read English. In such situations, it may be helpful for the patient's legal representative, having previously had the opportunity to discuss the matters with the patient with the assistance of an interpreter, to attend a CPA review and to put forward matters of concern on their behalf. In such a case, this would enable the solicitor acting for the patient to put forward the patient's concerns, for example, where reports in relation to their tribunal were only available to them in English and avoid seriously disadvantaging them in relation to instructing their solicitor. When this situation arose in a real case, it led to the hospital making arrangements for the reports to be translated into the patient's own language, which he was then able to read.

Despite the potential benefits to all those concerned, working together can have significant resource implications for clinical teams. Legal representatives and advocates will often tend to be proactive and not merely reactive. Particularly in the context of Mental Health Review Tribunal applications and the provision of aftercare, legal representatives will, from time to time, be required to involve other mental health care professionals to provide an independent assessment of clinical issues, specialist medicolegal matters, and aftercare and follow up arrangements.

Not infrequently, a patient's discharge from hospital may be delayed where their aftercare needs require the involvement of more than one form of service. Elderly patients suffering from mental illness, patients suffering from mental illness and learning disability, and patients with both physical and mental disabilities are some examples of how this situation can arise.

Case example 2

An elderly woman from a small ethnic minority group suffering from a severe form of physical illness as well as psychosis had been detained in hospital for a considerable period of time following the breakdown of a number of ethnically inappropriate community placements. The institution of MHRT proceedings, the indication of an intention to subpoena the director of social services and the health authority, and the threat of commencement of judicial review proceedings led to the allocation of the case to a mental health social worker. The use of an appropriately experienced independent social worker resolved the difficulty in identifying an ethnically appropriate and suitable placement. The prospect of the directors of social services and the health authority being required to attend the tribunal hearing also led to an early resolution of long outstanding funding issues. The long-term outcome of the identification of an ethnically appropriate placement was not only a very significant reduction in the patient's challenging behaviour but allowed the patient to fulfil a number of lifelong ambitions, not least of which was a visit to her homeland.

Delays can frequently be experienced with the Home Office in the granting of leave. In these circumstances, robust representation on the part of a patient's legal representative can often lead to expedition of decisions.

Case example 3

A patient had spent over 11 years in conditions of maximum security without making a great deal of progress towards movement to a less restrictive environment. When seen by an independent psychiatrist specialising in the treatment of personality disorder, it was suggested that the man might be suffering from Asperger's syndrome, a diagnosis subsequently confirmed by another independent psychiatrist specialising in the diagnosis and treatment of that particular condition. Acceptance of the diagnosis by the patient's clinical team led to a much clearer understanding of the reasons for the patient having not engaged in conventional rehabilitation programmes and shed fresh light on the appropriate way forward. The involvement of the independent psychiatrists and the making of the new diagnosis resulted from the involvement of the patient's solicitor.

For working together between the patient's clinical team and their legal representative or advocate to succeed, the members of the clinical team need to have a clear understanding of the role and obligations of the legal representative or advocate, a willingness to accommodate requests for information, and to provide opportunities for discussion and to cooperate with third-party experts where appropriate within the boundaries of normal professional behaviour and requirements, including in some instances, with due regard to the matter of confidentiality. They will also have to accept the need sometimes for the patient's legal representative or advocate to question decisions and put forward dissenting views.

Legal advocacy relates primarily not to the process of conducting or presenting a case before a court or tribunal, but in assisting users of mental health services to express themselves and to take an active part in the making of decisions affecting their lives. The assistance may sometimes take the form of speaking on behalf of the service user but will often also involve the provision of moral support to enable the individual to speak for himself or herself. Legal representatives, subject always to their client's instructions and the requirements of the Community Legal Service when publicly funded, have a duty to provide both representation and advice. That said, at present United Kingdom mental health legislation does not give any individual the right as such to advocacy and there is no statutory duty placed on authorities to ensure such provision. The National Service Framework for Mental Health (Department of Health, 1999) does nevertheless state that health authorities should have in place arrangements for the provision of advocacy services. This builds on The Patients Charter Implementation Guidance (Department of Health, 1997) that sets a basic standard for informing patients of any local advocacy schemes.

FUTURE MENTAL HEALTH LEGISLATION

The Draft Mental Health Bill 2002 for England and Wales (Department of Health, 2002) does place a duty on the appropriate Minister to make arrangements for the provision of an independent mental health advocacy service. It is proposed that help from mental health advocates must be made available to all patients who are subject to compulsory powers under Parts 2 or 3 of the Bill and to those who qualify for safeguards, such as patients with long-term incapacity under Part 5. If it passes into statute, advocates may also provide help to a patient's nominated person as defined in the Bill and intended as a replacement for the nearest relative, so long as the patient does not object. Provision will also be made for patients and their nominated person to be informed of their right to a mental health advocate at the time when compulsory powers are being put into effect. The type of help advocates will provide is set out and includes assistance in obtaining information about the medical treatment being provided, the legal authority under which treatment is being given and the patient's rights to challenge the use of compulsory powers to enforce such measures. Advocates will also help patients to exercise those rights, either by way of representation or otherwise and the explanatory notes which accompany the Draft Bill, give as an example 'by arranging legal advice for the patient'. The Bill provides that advocates will have a right to meet resident patients in private at any reasonable time. Advocates will also have the right to inspect any records relating to the patient and it will be unlawful for any person 'without reasonable cause' to prevent their access to the patients and/or their other records. The Bill allows the appropriate Minister to make regulations, setting out the standards that will need to be met by an individual in order to be approved as a mental health advocate.

In the accompanying explanatory notes (Department of Health, 2002), the government has indicated that 'The right to independent advocacy is drafted to comply with the positive duties imposed by Article 8 of the ECHR (European Convention of Human Rights) to ensure that mentally disordered persons are protected and have their rights to private life respected without interference, except as necessary in the interests of public safety or for the protection of the rights of others'.

THE ROLE OF ADVOCATES

In the absence currently of any nationally applicable standards for Legal Advocacy Services, most workers adopt the principle that their role is that of representation and information provision, and not the provision of legal advice or tribunal representation. If the law changes as it is proposed it should as described above, advocacy workers may have a far more important part to play in all patient care and certainly a much greater degree of formalisation of their role.

The United Kingdom Advocacy Network (NHS Executive, UKAN, 2000), in its code of practice, recommends that advocates do not take a deliberately adversarial stance, but neither do they seek to avoid confrontation and challenge when these are necessary. They seek to practise principled negotiation. Its guidance on the role of advocates suggests that:

- Advocates will only act or speak on the user's behalf as the user wishes.
- The key aim is to help people regain their own power and speak for themselves; advocates will support people when they speak for themselves.
- Advocates are there to speak with, rather than for people whenever possible. When it is not, they must take time to get to know the person and be very careful not to make assumptions based on their own preconceptions about what is good for them.

- People have an absolute right to be present when the advocate is discussing them.
- The advocate should make no decisions or choices on behalf of the service user.
- The advocate may discuss the various options with the service user in private and will attempt at all times to provide full and balanced information.
- It must be the service user who makes the decisions and choices whenever possible, even if the process of engagement is slow and uncertain.

As can be seen from this, the effective operation of advocacy services presents challenges for those involved as workers and clinical team members alike. An understanding of roles and fostering good interpersonal and professional relationships may be vital to the enhancement of the care of patients when mental health advocates are involved, particularly with detained longer term patients. One of the most difficult issues for both advocates and legal representatives is that of confidentiality. This inevitably also impacts upon the potential for good and fruitful relationships with the patient's clinical team and its individual members, whose professional parameters, in relation to the passage of patient information, may be different. In practice, the confidentiality policies of many advocacy schemes do not reflect the law. It is not widely appreciated how limited the protection given to confidential information is in general and in relation to medical matters, in particular. Generally, at common law, no privilege attaches to communications made in confidence, except to:

1. communications between a client and a legal advisor made for the purpose of the obtaining and giving of legal advice; and
2. communications between a client or his legal advisor and third parties, the dominant purpose of which was preparation for contemplated or pending litigation.

It follows that neither an advocate nor a legal representative, can give an absolute guarantee to a service user, that information will remain confidential. A legal advisor may be in a somewhat stronger position.

UKAN in its code of practice provides that:

- Advocates will disclose to service users complete details of all communications concerning them, but they will not disclose information about them to others without their express consent.
- Staff should make relevant information available to the advocate (with the person's permission) and should be aware that an advocate will always share any given information with that person.
- An advocate should not sign any statement that allows the advocate to know, or keep confidential from the person, details of clinical history or treatment.

The 'Guide to professional conduct of solicitors' (Law Society, 1999) advises that they may reveal confidential information to the extent that the solicitor believes it necessary, to prevent the client or a third party committing a criminal act that the solicitor believes on reasonable grounds is likely to result in serious bodily harm.

A study commissioned by the Department of Health (Barnes et al., 2002) in its recommendations for good practice stated that:

- Specialist advocacy is independent professional advocacy for individuals who are subject to the powers of mental health legislation in England and Wales.
- The model of advocacy proposed is that of professional advocacy—a service provided by trained paid advocates. Volunteers may make a valuable contribution and add value to the service, but paid employees should provide the core specialist work.

It also recommended core standards for independent specialist advocacy (Independent Specialist Advocacy in England and Wales, 2002), including those relating to service principles largely in keeping with the existing UKAN code of practice and providing that 'confidentiality should only be broken when a service user threatens to harm him/her self or others'.

Amongst the recommended 'Responsibilities of service providers' are that all staff should be informed and trained on the principles of advocacy, staff and advocates should work together to develop good quality, user friendly, information about advocacy, and staff should ensure advocates can attend meetings at the request of service users whose care and treatment will be discussed. The advocate should be informed even if a meeting is called at short notice.

The majority of legal representatives, but not all, will be members of the Law Society's specialist Mental Health Review Tribunal Panel and work for a firm of solicitors holding a Legal Services Commission Mental Health Franchise. Mental health advice and representation are provided under the terms of a General Civil Contract between the individual firm and the Legal Services Commission and fall into two categories:

1. *controlled legal representation*, which can be provided to a client in proceedings before a Mental Health Review Tribunal under the Mental Health Act 1983, where the clients case or application to the tribunal is or is to be the subject of those proceedings and which can be provided without reference to the client's financial resources, but should not be provided where it is unreasonable to do so in the particular circumstances of the case; and
2. *legal help*, but not representation, which can be provided for mental health and community care-related matters that are not the subject of present or prospective tribunal proceedings. Legal help is subject to both a means and merits test, in accordance with detailed criteria set out in the Legal Services Commission Funding Code (The Legal Services Commission Manual, 2003a) and Decision Making Guidance (The Legal Services Commission Manual, 2003b).

Both types of assistance are subject in individual matters to overall financial limits set by the Legal Services Commission.

GUIDELINES FOR LEGAL REPRESENTATIVES AND PANEL MEMBERS

Membership of the Law Society's specialist Mental Health Review Tribunal Panel is subject to attendance on a qualifying course and a successful assessment. The Law Society provides guidelines for legal representatives and panel members. Panel members are required to sign an undertaking that they will not normally delegate the preparation, supervision, conduct or presentation of a case, but will deal with it personally. The guidelines provide that, whilst it is the patients' views or wishes that should be represented to a tribunal and that a legal representative should act in accordance with the patient's instructions, solicitors have a general duty at all times to act in the best interests of the client. This includes a requirement to give clients their best advice, which in MHRT cases might include a realistic assessment of the likelihood of the patient being discharged or advice on possible steps towards discharge. That said, the client, of course, has the right not to accept that advice. The guidance further recognises that some patients detained under the Act (Mental Health Act 1983) will not have the mental capacity to give clear instructions to their solicitor and provides that it can generally be assumed that, in applying to the MHRT, the patient is asking the Tribunal to review the grounds for their compulsory detention under the Mental Health Act, since that is the purpose of the MHRT.

In relation to automatic references and patients who lack capacity, the guidance states that the Law Society takes the view that it is not appropriate to appoint a next friend or guardian *ad litem*, since the patient has neither made the application nor are they defending the proceedings, as the MHRT proceedings were started by process rather than by application. The guidance goes on to say that a solicitor asked by the tribunal office or by hospital managers to represent the patient in such cases is not instructed by the tribunal or the managers, but is in fact acting without instructions.

In the specific context of the MHRT rules 6 and 12 (MHRT Rules, 1983), which deal with information not to be disclosed, provide a statutory exception to the legal representatives' obligation of disclosure of information to their client.

The European Court and Commission has established the need to protect the interests of persons who, on account of their mental disabilities, are not fully capable of acting for themselves, where necessary, through some form of representation. In particular, Article 5(4) does not require individuals detained under Article 5(1)(e) to take the initiative in obtaining legal advice and representation (Convention for the Protection of Human Rights and Fundamental Freedoms, 1950).

In Winterwerp v Netherlands, the European Commission said that the patient's lawyer had the right to examine the patient's file (European Commission of Human Rights). In Aerts v Belgium (1998), the ECHR held that the right to liberty is a civil right within Article 6(1) (right to a fair trial) (Convention for the Protection of Human Rights and Fundamental Freedoms, 1950).

In Re: L (Care: Assessment: fair trial; 2002), Munby J held:

- The right to a fair trial in Article 6 of the Convention was not confined to the purely judicial part of the proceedings. Unfairness at any stage of the litigation process might involve breaches not merely of Article 8 but also of Article 6.

• Crucial meetings, at which a family's future was being decided, must be conducted openly and with the parents if they wished either present or represented.
• Documents produced at, and minutes of, meetings should be made available to those who attended them, including family members.

The latter case has, by analogy, implications in relation to MHRT proceedings, which engage both Article 8 and Article 6.

CONCLUDING REMARKS

Both advocates and legal representatives, by seeking to work with a patient's clinical team, can contribute significantly to improved communication and a sense of greater involvement on the part of the patient. The role of the advocate, particularly the proposed new specialist advocate, is likely to be more circumscribed than that of the legal representative, especially in the context of MHRTs in relation to aftercare arrangements. Close liaison between the patient's clinical and legal team can, in certain circumstances, lead to a pooling of resources, enabling the targeted use of independent experts and, in extreme cases, the tactical use of complaints and judicial review proceedings, to the benefit of the patient. In order for patients' legal representatives and advocates to be able to work together effectively with the patient's clinical team, it is important that hospitals have policies and guidance in place, covering amongst other matters, access to records, information sharing, confidentiality, attendance at meetings and a wide range of other issues.

Within the appropriate legal framework, practice guidelines and clinical approaches, therefore, there may be, it can be argued, a variety of ways in which advocates and legal representatives can work with, if not as part of, a clinical team, to enhance the care and management of patients and clients. This is arguably particularly the case when patients are detained in hospital on a compulsory basis and especially for those subject to more restrictive forms of compulsory care. Nevertheless, this working relationship requires work, tolerance and an understanding of roles and professional boundaries. While clinicians need to be able to accept challenges to their approach or decisions, the patient's legal representative must avoid any apparent loss of the independence that is so important and central to their work with and for the mentally disordered individual.

References

Aerts v Belgium [1998] EHRLR 777

Barnes D, Brandon T and Webb T (2002) Independent specialist advocacy in England and Wales: recommendations for good practice. Core standards. Department of Health and University of Durham. London: HMSO

Convention for the Protection of Human Rights and Fundamental Freedoms (1950) Strasbourg: Council of Europe

Department of Health (1997) The patients charter and mental health services implementation guidance. London: HMSO

Department of Health (1999) Mental health national service framework: modern standards and service models. London: HMSO

Department of Health (2002) Draft Mental Health Bill explanatory notes. London: HMSO

European Commission of Human Rights Application No 6301/73

Law Society (1999) The guide to professional conduct of solicitors. London: Law Society

Law Society Representation at Mental Health Review Tribunals Guidelines for Legal Representatives (1983) London: Law Society

Legal Services Commission Manual (2003a) Access to Justice Act 1999, Vol. 3. London: Sweet and Maxwell

Legal Services Commission Manual (2003b) The funding code, decision making guidance, Vol. 3. London: Sweet and Maxwell

Mental Health Act 1983. London: HMSO

Mental Health Tribunal Rules 1983. London: HMSO

MHRT Rules (1983) Statutory guidance. No 942. London: HMSO

NHS Executive Mental Health Task Force User Group UKAN (United Kingdom Advocacy Network) (2002) Advocacy: a code of practice. London: HMSO

NHSE Circular EL(97)1 16.1.97

Re: L (Care Assessment: Fair Trial) [2002] EWHC 1379 [2002] 2 FLR 730

Chapter **5**

Specific joint working II: The ideal and reality of multidisciplinary working in prisons

Luke Birmingham, Carol Peckham and Vincent Baxter

INTRODUCTION

Multidisciplinary working with mentally disordered offenders in community and hospital settings can be fraught with problems, and is particularly the case when trying to adopt this model with prisoners. This section considers the reality and the ideal of multidisciplinary working in prisons, and explores some of the obstacles to effective multidisciplinary and multiagency working there and examines ways of overcoming some of these barriers.

THE PRISON SYSTEM IN ENGLAND AND WALES

Many prisons in use today were originally built in the mid to late 1800s when imprisonment replaced execution and transportation as the principal means of dealing with people convicted of serious offences. Despite refurbishment and an extensive building programme, the prison estate relies heavily on old stock that is not fit for a modern-day prison service (Prison Service, 2000a).

There are currently 138 prisons in England and Wales. Variations in size, location, function, culture and design mean that each institution is unique. Prisons can be classified according to the highest security category of prisoner they can accommodate. There are four of these categories: A, B, C and D. Category A applies to prisoners for whom escape must be made virtually impossible because of the danger they would pose if at large. Category B applies to prisoners for whom the very highest conditions of security are not necessary, but for whom escape must be made very difficult. Category C applies to those who cannot be trusted in open conditions, but who do not have the resources or the will to make a determined attempt to escape. Category D applies to prisoners who can reasonably be trusted in open conditions.

Security is the primary concern of the Prison Service (2000b) and, as such, it overshadows every other aspect of prison life. The Prison Service relies on a combination of regimes and strict rules to promote good order and discipline, and maintain security. Regimes regulate the activity of prisoners from reception to discharge and rules govern daily operations in the institution (Prison Service, 2000b).

Prisons are known to overestimate the amount of time spent by prisoners out of their cells, and activities that are provided do not always meet prisoner's needs or help them develop skills they can use after their release. This is a particular problem in local prisons, where some inmates are locked up as long as 23 hours a day. In some training prisons, only a third of prisoners report being involved in some kind of training or education (Her Majesty's (HM) Inspectorate of Prisons, 2000, 2002).

THE PRISON POPULATION

The prison population in England and Wales has risen steadily over the last decade. In 2001, the average population in custody stood at 66 300, an increase of 45% compared to 1991. By the end of 2002, the prison population had risen to over 72 000 (Home Office, 2002, 2003). The Prison Service has struggled to cope with the growth in prisoner numbers and many establishments are overcrowded as a result. In 2001, nearly one in five prisoners were doubled up with two people sharing cells designed for one (Home Office, 2003).

Prisoners are a transient population. There are more than 140 000 new receptions into prisons in England and Wales each year (Department of Health, 2001). Most of those who are remanded into custody spend less than 6 weeks in prison. Three-quarters of offenders who receive a prison sentence are given 2 years or less. Taking into account time served on remand and release provisions, this means that more than four-fifths of all sentenced prisoners are released within 12 months of sentencing. Half of those released will be reconvicted within 2 years (HM Inspectorate of Prisons, 2001; Home Office 2003).

Abuse during childhood, deprivation, homelessness, unemployment, substance misuse and mental health problems are commonplace among people in prison. A large proportion of them have problems with numeracy and literacy, and most prisoners are below average intelligence (HM Inspectorate of Prisons, 1997, 2000; Singleton et al., 1998).

The prevalence of psychiatric morbidity is much higher among people in prison than in the general population. A recent systematic review of serious mental disorder among prisoners found that about one in seven prisoners in Westernised countries have a psychotic illness or major depression, and about one in two men and one in five women in prison have antisocial personality disorder (Fazel and Danesh, 2000). A comprehensive survey of psychiatric morbidity among prisoners in England

and Wales was carried out in 1997 on behalf of the Office for National Statistics. This study, which screened prisoners for five categories of mental disorder, namely psychotic illness, neurotic conditions, personality disorder, hazardous drinking and drug dependence, found very high rates of mental abnormality. Less than one in ten prisoners interviewed showed no evidence at all of mental disorder. In excess of seven out of ten had disorders from two or more of the above categories (Singleton et al., 1998). Self-harm is prevalent and the suicide rate among prisoners remains high (Prison Service, 2001). A very high proportion of those interviewed during the 1997 national prison survey said that they had thought about committing suicide at some point (Singleton et al., 1998). Twelve per cent of male remand prisoners said they had experienced suicidal thoughts in the week prior to interview and 15% said they had attempted suicide in the previous year (Singleton et al., 1998).

The Office for National Statistics prison survey also found that 18% of male sentenced prisoners, 21% of male remand prisoners and 40% of women prisoners said they had been receiving help for mental or emotional problems in the year prior to coming into prison (Singleton et al., 1998). Twenty-two per cent of female remand prisoners said they had been admitted to a psychiatric hospital at some point in their lives, including 6% who were inpatients for 6 months or more and 11% who had been admitted to a locked ward.

PRISON HEALTH CARE

The report by the Joint Prison Service and National Health Service (NHS) Executive Working Group (HM Prison Service and NHS Executive, 1999) states that 'health care in prisons is characterised by considerable variation in organisation and delivery, quality, funding and effectiveness, and links with the NHS'. The report views the situation as largely the product of the historical and *ad hoc* development of the prison health care system. Prison health services have been something of a neglected issue according to the Prison Health Policy Unit and Task Force (Department of Health and HM Prison Service, 2001), often afforded low priority by a Prison Service under pressure to cope with a growing inmate population and deliver greater efficiency. The service has also tended to operate in relative isolation from the NHS and, combined with a regime that is firmly structured and organised, with a traditional hierarchy of roles and system of rules, rewards and punishments, the prison environment provides a challenge to all those who choose to deliver health care within it.

The delivery of health care within Prisons in the United Kingdom falls mainly on health care staff and teams. These are comprised of a mixture of Prison Service staff, for instance, Prison Service nurses and health care officers, and NHS staff, for instance, community psychiatric nurses and psychiatrists. Together they deliver care to a population made up disproportionately of men who drink and smoke heavily, have far more active health problems than the population at large, and show evidence of self-neglect (United Kingdom Central Council for Nursing, Midwifery and Health Visiting, 1999).

Working with a population that has complex health and social care needs within a highly restrictive environment raises many issues. It requires approaches that respect the rights and needs of individuals, whilst at the same time maintaining a system that is safe and secure. Through exploration of these issues and approaches, a picture of day-to-day working within prison can be built up, and the impact this has upon those who deliver health care and those who receive it.

The Health Care Service for prisoners, formerly known as the Prison Medical Service, is Britain's oldest civilian medical service (Smith, 1983). This small, isolated and under-resourced organisation has been repeatedly criticised for providing prisoners with inferior health care (Smith, 1999). An opportunity to integrate prison medicine into mainstream health care was created when the NHS was founded in 1948, but the move was rejected and the two organisations remained separate until very recently. In 2000, the NHS entered into a health care partnership with the Prison Service. As a result, the NHS has taken over responsibility for secondary health care in prisons but, according to the Prisons Act 1952, for the moment, the overall responsibility for the care of people in prison still rests with the Home Secretary and the Prison Service.

The Prison Medical Service had its origins in the 1774 Prison Act for preserving the health of prisoners (Sim, 1990). The service was in a ramshackle state until the mid-1800s, when new convict prisons were built to accommodate the expanding population, new regulations for the appointment of prison doctors were introduced and the entire prison system came under central government control (Hardy, 1995). These changes brought about a more organised prison medical service, but they did not benefit the hordes of prisoners with physical and mental health problems. The reason for this relates to the fact that the main duty of the prison doctor was to provide regular reports to the prison authorities on the health of prisoners, rather than individual or other treatments. Doctors also became involved in more ethically unsound practices, such as the supervision of punishment, using unspeakable methods to identify feigned insanity and manipulating prisoners' diets to improve moral health (Sim, 1990). These institutional legacies can still be seen in prisons today. A prison doctor can authorise segregation on medical grounds, may determine whether prisoners are fit for adjudication or punishment, and are expected to try the food before it is served. Another characteristic of prison medicine is its reluctance to part with the traditional medically led model of health. Psychologists have been employed in prisons since the 1930s, but their work, which concentrates on reducing offending behaviour, is largely separate from health care. Nurses have only recently been introduced into prisons. Before this, the only other non-managerial health care staff were hospital officers, discipline officers with rudimentary health care training, whose main function was to assist the prison doctor.

The traditional model of prison health care that still exists in many prisons today focuses on screening new prisoners for health problems at reception and delivering services from the prison health care centre. Studies looking at the traditional method of reception health screening have shown this to be cursory and ineffective (Mitchinson et al., 1994; Birmingham et al., 1997; Parsons et al., 2001). Most new prisoners with mental disorder were missed at reception. This resulted in them being placed on ordinary prison wings where their problems remained undetected. On prison wings, the expectation has always been that prisoners will report sick to see a doctor in the health care centre. As a result, those with severe mental health problems tend to be overlooked, unless they cause considerable disruption and become a management problem, in which case staff may refer them for medical assessment.

Health care provision varies considerably from prison to prison. Larger, more secure institutions tend to have health care centres with 24-hour, staffed, inpatient beds. They provide this form of cover for a cluster of neighbouring prisons. This means that a category C or D prisoner, who needs 24-hour prison inpatient care, has to be transferred to a more secure institution with a more restrictive regime. Elsewhere, although they are commonly referred to as hospitals, prison health care centres are more like sick bays with primary health care facilities only. The Mental Health Act does not apply to inpatient care in prisons. This means that treatment for mental disorder cannot be given without a prisoner's consent unless there is justification for doing so under common law. Prisoners with serious mental health problems who require compulsory treatment have to be transferred to outside hospitals for this.

In many prisons, health care beds are included in the certified normal accommodation (CNA) quota. This means that when the prison is full, health care centre beds are used as 'ordinary' cells to accommodate prisoners who do not need to be there. Prisoners with mental health problems occupy most of the 1700 beds that are provided in prison health care centres. Reed and Lyne (1997, 2000) found that the mentally ill prisoners they studied faced lengthy waits for NHS beds and, whilst in prison, they spent long periods of time locked up and in seclusion. They also found that prison health care was often of low quality: staff were inadequately trained and supported to do their work and occupational therapy and clinical psychology input was scarce. Specialist health care for prisoners with mental health problems is still provided in many cases by visiting NHS psychiatrists, employed on a sessional basis. This usually offers little more than a fire-fighting service.

The prison health care system has continually been criticised for failing to provide NHS-equivalent standards. Most recently, conditions in some health care centres were described by Martin Narey, Director General of the Prison Service for England and Wales, as 'worse than the kennels I leave my dog in when I go on holiday' (Tucker, 2001). However, since prison health care operates within an environment with a strong emphasis on security rather than health improvement, such criticism may seem harsh. Time constraints, and the strict guidelines health care staff are expected to work to, often limit the type and quality of service they are able to provide. For example, it is reported that such factors can have a significant impact upon health screening procedures at first reception, where they can affect the quality of information obtained from prisoners and the response to important findings (Mitchison et al., 1994).

This failure to detect and respond to health issues adequately impacts in a number of ways, such as influencing location within the prison and subsequent access to treatment.

JOINT WORKING IN PRISONS: THE REALITY

People who are remanded or sentenced to prison will be dealt with by the police, courts, the Prison Service, including discipline officers, governors and prison health care staff, the Probation Service and, as a matter of course, may also come into contact with staff contracted to provide education, professionals who deliver offender treatment programmes, health care staff employed by the NHS, social services, drug and alcohol services, the Church, other religious organisations, and voluntary sector services. The police, courts and the Prison Service are particularly concerned with public protection. This is probably also true of today's probation service. Other agencies have different objectives, with staff tending to place more emphasis on addressing the unmet needs of prisoners than security. In order to achieve the correct balance between security and meeting prisoners' needs, all of the agencies concerned have to develop effective methods of joint working. Unfortunately, there is still little evidence that this type of approach is being adopted in prisons. One of the main reasons for this is the lack of understanding of the framework, ethos and priorities within which other agencies operate (Shakespeare, 2000). Other barriers include different values, mismatched organisational structures and diverse professional cultures (Webb, 1991), as well as the pessimism with which prisoners with mental health problems are viewed by health, social services, and the Probation Service and Prison Service (Harris, 1999).

Over the last 20 years, the courts, prisons and the Probation Service have been trying to establish 'what works' in sentencing. Sentence planning was introduced in order to address offending behaviour more systematically and achieve 'seamless sentences', before and after release. However, the recent preoccupation with security by the Prison Service and the Probation Service's focus on the risk of harm to others has meant that work on the resettlement of prisoners, which aims to reintegrate them effectively back into the community, has been sadly neglected (HM Inspectorate of Prisons, 2001). The situation is made worse by the fact that there is no national strategy. The Government has published a National Correctional Policy Framework, which highlights the need to build effective partnerships and liaison between agencies involved with offenders, and to develop effective mechanisms of information exchange, accurate methods of risk assessment, and accredited offender treatment programmes (Home Office, 1999). However, achieving these objectives will require fundamental changes in the culture and procedures of the Prison Service and the Probation Service.

Committal into custody removes an individual from their normal environment. This separation also dislocates them from any existing support network and compromises coping mechanisms. Therefore, the Prison Service has a duty of care to ensure that adequate means of support exists in order to sustain vulnerable prisoners and enable them to deal with the burden of custody. To this end, the Prison Service, and in particular health care staff, have adopted approaches that seek to assess risk and prevent suicide and self-harm specifically.

If an individual is identified as being at risk of suicide/self-harm, then a purpose-designed file called an F2052SH can be opened. This document is issued by HM Prison Service and came into operation on 1 April 1994, its aim being to enable high-quality care to be given to vulnerable individuals through positive, effective, communication between all staff and agencies involved with the individual concerned through the provision of a detailed plan of support. This is intended not only to provide support to the prisoner but also the staff, since it requires all those in contact with the particular inmate to share in the process of care and management. Occasionally, an individual may be identified as being in need of constant support or a place of safety to help them during a time of crisis. Location in a multicell or crisis suite where the inmate is never left alone, being placed on constant watch or within an antiligature cell are all practical steps that can be taken in order to facilitate this.

However, interventions are also required that not only manage the risk of suicide and self-harm, but also affect the underlying problems. Collaboration between all those working within the prison environment can ensure that mental disorder, a factor linked to self-harm and completed suicide, is recognised and treated appropriately. Programmes focusing on problem-solving, social skills and assertiveness training can address some deficits that are recognised as being present in some individuals who become involved in episodes of self-harm (Macleod et al., 1992).

It is interesting to note that the Offender Assessment System (OASys), which has recently been introduced to assess the likelihood of reoffending as well as the risks that an individual poses to themselves and others, includes aspects of health (National Probation Service, 2002). At present, OASys only involves the Probation Service and Prison Service. It does not incorporate formal input from health or social services. Sharing information and breaching confidentiality may be a potential problem. However, it is important to bear in mind that many of the homicide inquiries, carried out on individuals in previous contact with mental health services who have killed, have stressed the need for better communication and sharing of information between agencies (Reith, 1998). The situation is hindered by information-sharing protocols and information technology systems in prisons that are woefully inadequate. It is also compounded by the fact that agencies that work with prisoners have little knowledge or understanding of the assessment tools employed by other professionals who are working alongside them.

As far as health care is concerned, it is clear that the historical legacy left by the Prison Medical Service serves to reinforce many of the barriers that already exist in prisons to develop more effective methods of joint working. The Prison Service admits that prison health care is over-medicalised. It is reactive rather than proactive and is characterised by lack of direction, poor communication and confused lines of accountability. It places more emphasis on process than outcome (HM Prison Service and NHS Executive, 1999).

Imprisoning individuals with mental health problems can present a number of problems. It can worsen the situation in certain circumstances, lead to relapse and re-emergence of symptoms and prevent mentally ill individuals from receiving the treatment they require. Long waiting lists for NHS beds mean that those individuals who are assessed as needing transfer to hospital for treatment have to be cared for in less than ideal conditions. Mentally ill prisoners refusing treatment can often remain untreated because, under current mental health legislation, prison hospitals are classified as a 'place of safety' and, as such, medication and other forms of treatment must only be used with appropriate consent and may not be enforced. Prisoners in contact with psychiatric services prior to their detention can often lose contact with clinicians previously involved in their care. In a recent study about their role in the care of inmates they had been in contact with prior to their admission to prison, 25% of adult consultant psychiatrists reported never being made aware of the individual's detention, while a further 42% estimated they were informed less than half the time (Smith et al., 2002).

The prison health care experience need not, however, be a negative one. The fact that prisoners are clearly a 'captive audience' provides an opportunity for those caring for them to tackle the vast array of health and social care needs and problems that this group present. Nevertheless, this is not an easy task, given the mixed bag of disciplines and agencies working within the prison environment, and the fact that each one may have a primary allegiance to delivering health and social care or maintaining discipline and security.

According to the Prison Inspectorate, prison health care services have little commitment to or understanding of a planned, coordinated approach for the delivery of health care to prisoners (HM Inspectorate of Prisons, 1996). The Prison Health Service has also functioned in relative isolation for many years with few ties to the NHS. The separate system used for keeping health records in prison provides a good example of the sort of problems that this way of working creates. The inmate medical record (IMR), a file that is opened on every new prisoner, does not routinely contain any information from the prisoner's NHS records. If this is required, it must be requested by the prison doctor. There may be considerable delays in obtaining this information from general practitioners (GPs) and hospital medical record departments. Some are reluctant to provide the information and GPs may wish to charge for the service. When the prisoner is released, the IMR is archived. Because it is not routine practice to correspond with the GP or mental health services, continuity of care is almost impossible to achieve. Worse still, since there is no system for tracking or storage of IMRs, if the individual concerned is imprisoned again at a future date, it is likely that they will have a new IMR opened, whilst their old records remain in storage (Health Advisory Committee, 1997).

Joint working in prison is also hampered by staff shortages, low morale and overcrowding. These problems place considerable strains on the day-to-day running of establishments and, as a result, it can be hard for staff to find the time and motivation to pursue complex tasks.

Cultural factors are also a major obstacle to change. It is still the case that most staff working in prison health care are employed by the Prison Service. There are more qualified nurses working in prisons than previously, but the Prison Service still employs non-nursing qualified health care officers, who are essentially prison officers who have undergone basic health care training to deliver health care. This creates role ambiguity for staff and differing line management structures, resulting in confused accountability (HM Prison Service and NHS Executive, 2000). Prisons continue to have difficulties recruiting and retaining suitably qualified health care staff, and the fact that continuing professional development for staff has not been well established is an ongoing source of concern (HM Prison Service and NHS Executive, 1999; Tucker, 2001).

The Care Programme Approach (CPA) (Department of Health, 1990) is widely used in the community to address the complex needs of mentally disordered offenders. The framework of the CPA, which is grounded in the principles of multidisciplinary working and user involvement, is now being used in hospital inpatient and community care settings but it is not routinely applied in prisons. According to Shaw (2002), in the few prisons where it has been introduced, it has been implemented in an *ad hoc* fashion with little or no attempt to evaluate its effectiveness. Perhaps the main reason why CPA has not been used more widely in prisons is that the NHS was not accountable for prisoners until very recently. However, problems with implementing CPA in prison probably also reflects the fact that providing effective, well-coordinated care in a secure setting, where health care is a matter of secondary importance, is very difficult (Dale and Woods, 2002). This was certainly evident when the process of CPA was analysed in a local remand prison (Lart, 1997), where participants focused more on their roles and boundaries, and had less understanding of the range of tasks that need to be allocated and completed.

THERAPY VERSUS SECURITY

Prison health care staff work within a unique environment and face the problem of being viewed by the inmates as being responsible for both therapy and security. This may result in many prisoners mistrusting health care workers or refusing to use the facilities available to improve their health (Walsh, 1998). Health care professionals visiting prisons are faced with an environment and culture that can often lead to difficult behaviour being interpreted as a discipline-related issue rather than a possible symptom of an illness requiring therapeutic intervention. In addition, staff may be wary of showing sympathy to distressed individuals.

Prison health care staff and clinicians, while striving to uphold the best possible standards of care and professionalism, must do so while maintaining safety and security. The role of the health care officer is intended to combine the approaches of discipline and health care needs. This is a difficult balance to maintain, and the success or otherwise of the post may come down to the individual and their personal characteristics and approach. Prison nursing staff are often required to carry out non-nursing tasks, such as escorting prisoners and, over time, many begin to adopt the disciplinary approach. Many prison nurses report feeling that their obligations to being professionally accountable are compromised by the environment in which they operate (Tucker, 2001). They also describe a sense of professional isolation.

For those health care professionals visiting prisons, the strict disciplinary lines along which the institution is run can be frustrating and impede the work they are attempting to carry out. They can also face perceived or actual pressures to compromise their standards from those within the Prison Service who fail to understand or recognise their professional obligations. The tension between the health care needs of prisoners and those of the establishment relating primarily to security and control can result in scepticism on the part of inmates towards health care staff, and can lead to the questioning of their motives and actions. Mistrust can also work in the opposite direction, and health care staff need to be alert to the fact that some prisoners may attempt to exploit certain situations in order to undermine security procedures. For example, hospital appointments outside of the prison can provide an opportunity for escape.

Security and therapy are issues that cannot be separated. Aspects of both need to be integrated into the care of prisoners, something that has been achieved reasonably successfully within forensic mental health care settings. The rights of prisoners should perhaps only be limited if the exercise of them unnecessarily compromises their own security, or fails to take reasonable account of the rights and security requirements of others.

COMPETING CULTURES

If a modern approach to prison health care is to evolve, then the cultural differences that currently exist within prisons must be tackled. Many of these originate from a lack of knowledge about the roles of the different professions involved, traditional interdisciplinary and interagency suspicions, statutory duties and prison rules, and the inevitable resistance to change that bedevils every organisation.

Historically, health care in prisons has been developed within the service as an element of the overall regime, and as a consequence has led to the development of a number of problematic issues. For example, there is often pressure on prison health centres with inpatient facilities to operate at 100% occupancy resulting in the non-clinical use of health care accommodation on occasions as already described. The frequent use of prison health centres to manage prisoners who fail to cope on the prison wings and for whom social support rather than medical care would be more appropriate is a clear example of this fact.

Interactions between various individuals and groups within prisons can also have a significant impact upon the way health care is delivered. The most notable are those that occur between custody staff and the various groups delivering health care. For example, it has been reported that some custody staff seem to view inmate health care as a distraction and an interference with the performance of their own duties, while others consider it to be of benefit, not only to inmates but also themselves in the undertaking of their own work (Droes, 1994).

While acknowledging that, within prisons, therapy and security cannot be viewed in isolation, there is perhaps some scope for overcoming the care versus custody dilemma by separating out or revising the two roles. In Northern Ireland, for instance, the Prison Service employs registered nurses as nurse officers. These staff have a dual role in both health and discipline fields, but only within health care settings or related situations. They cannot be deployed to carry out general discipline duties. This enables them to integrate into the prison culture without any apparent difficulties (Tucker, 2001). In Scottish prisons, only nurses work within health care, alongside other health professionals, thus dispensing with the traditional health care officer role. This has resulted in Scottish prison health care becoming nurse-led and, therefore, allowing it to become an integral part of sentence management (Tucker, 2001).

Prison custody staff can exert significant influence over health care, while nurses working within the prison environment who have increased levels of education and experience can provide a broader scope of health care to inmates (Droes, 1994). If the traditional wariness and scepticism that exists between these two groups can be overcome and can be coupled with the empowerment of nursing staff, then more favourable conditions for health care delivery in prisons may begin to develop.

WORKING IN PARTNERSHIP

The need for the provision of both appropriate and comprehensive health services for prisoners has been recognised for some time now and publicised by the production of a number of influential reports (Home Office, 1990; Department of Health and Home Office, 1992). These have not only highlighted the state of prison health care, but also provided the catalyst for new service provision to be planned, providing a political edge to a neglected area of penal reform. Funding for new initiatives became accessible and various schemes, including those aimed at diverting individuals with mental health problems away from the criminal justice system and into the health care system, have been developed. Prison diversion, or remand liaison schemes, are examples of the many different services that have evolved in response to the call for health care to be improved within the criminal justice system. The nature of these schemes has tended to depend upon local determining factors, such as the maturity of interagency relations, collaborative intent and the availability of NHS facilities. As a consequence, each tends to be different in the type of service it offers. Examples are those that exist at HM Prisons Birmingham, Exeter and Belmarsh. However, despite the many differences between the different services that have evolved, they each rely on partnership with the prison concerned to make it work. While many NHS professionals have the therapeutic skills necessary for delivering care, they often lack the specialist skills acquired by staff working in custodial settings.

FUTURE DEVELOPMENTS

The past decade has seen the growth and development of many local diversion schemes. However, this era may now be coming to an end. Research has shown that the complex nature of the problems presented by mentally disordered individuals who come into contact with the criminal justice system cannot be met by small schemes that are often isolated from mainstream services. Future services, it is suggested, will need to adopt a more integrated multiagency approach, be properly coordinated at both local and national level, and be provided with adequate resources (Birmingham, 2001).

These first steps, aimed at providing better and more integrated health services for prisoners, represent a significant change in the way prison health care is delivered. However, it should be recognised that many operational and cultural differences exist both within and between the Prison Service and the NHS, and both services need to acknowledge the particular skills, resources and experiences each has to offer. The key to the future delivery of health care in prisons lies in linking the potential each service has to offer and forging it into an effective partnership capable of delivering tangible change.

THE WAY FORWARD

Support for developing multidisciplinary and multiagency models of working in prison is gathering momentum, and changes in policy resulting from modern-day reform of prison health care is beginning to have an impact on the standards and delivery of health care to prisoners. Although the Prison Service has openly acknowledged for a decade or more that prisoners should have access to the same quality and range of health care services as the general public receives from the NHS (Prison Service, 1994), the current reform of prison health care really only began to take shape after the government established a joint NHS Executive and Prison Service working party to consider recommendations made by the Chief Inspector of Prisons in a discussion document entitled 'Patient or prisoner?' (HM Inspectorate of Prisons, 1996). The Chief Inspector recommended that responsibility for providing health care to prisoners should be transferred from the Prison Service to the NHS. The joint working party report, published in 1999, endorsed the principle of equivalence of care, but the suggestion that the NHS should assume full responsibility for prison health care was rejected. Instead, the working party recommended establishing a joint partnership between the Prison Service and the NHS, with the former being largely responsible for primary care and the NHS taking over responsibility for secondary care. What this meant was that the NHS would no longer be able to relinquish responsibility for patients at the prison gate (HM Prison Service and NHS Executive, 1999).

The recommendation to establish a health care partnership between the NHS and the Prison Service, which ministers accepted, has resulted in a considerable amount of organisational change in the last few years. At a national level, the Home Office directorate of prison health care was dissolved and, in April 2000, two new bodies, the Prison Health Policy Unit and Task Force, were created. The Task Force and the Policy Unit report jointly to the Home Office and the Department of Health to help ensure that NHS and Prison Service policies complement each other. One of their principal aims is to work together to coordinate the development of mental health services in prisons. At a local level, prisons and local NHS partners have begun to identify and meet the health care needs of those in prison.

The principle of equivalence of care means that plans to modernise services for mentally disordered prisoners have to be developed in line with NHS mental health policy and the National Service Framework for mental health (Department of Health, 1999). The NHS Plan makes a commitment to employing 300 extra staff to provide mental health services for prisoners. It also states that:

> by 2004, 5000 prisoners at any one time should be receiving more comprehensive mental health services in prison. All people with severe mental illness will be in receipt of treatment, and no prisoner with serious mental illness will leave prison without a care plan or a care co-ordinator.
>
> (Department of Health, 2000)

In order to deliver on the NHS Plan and ensure that improvements in prison health care services comply with standards set out in the National Service Framework for mental health, the Department of Health and the Prison Service have jointly identified a number of themes. These are promoting mental health, primary care services, wing-based services; day care services; inpatient services; transfer to NHS facilities; through care, access to effective treatments and suicide prevention (Department of Health, 2001). The idea is that these themes will be underpinned by the principles of multidisciplinary working and effective collaboration between different agencies.

Mental health promotion emphasises the need for mental health awareness training for prison officers so they can recognise prisoners who may be in need of more intensive support and/or possible referral to the specialist services. Primary care services in prisons should mirror primary care in the general community. This includes being able to identify and refer prisoners with more complex mental health problems without delay so that appropriate advice on management and treatment can be given. Reception screening is an important aspect of this in order to avoid delay in access to treatment. Wing-based services are about providing support and treatment for prisoners with mental health problems in the main residential areas of establishments rather than automatically transferring them to the prison health care centre. This means that, wherever possible, anyone entering prison with an existing CPA care plan should have this continued in 'normal' surroundings with the help and support of prison staff. Again, training would be beneficial to optimise the level of care that can be offered. More intensive support will be provided by means of day care services. The intention is to enable clinical psychologists, occupational therapists and other specialist staff to provide treatment in a way that allows prisoners to continue to make use of existing facilities, such as gym and education, but also provide specific therapy alongside existing regimes. It is hoped that the introduction of these measures will reduce the pressure on prison health care centre beds as these beds should be reserved for the minority of prisoners who need 24-hour support and supervision.

For those with serious mental health problems who are inappropriately placed in prison, transfer to NHS facilities must be high priority. This will require active engagement with all staff both from the receiving unit and the referring establishment. Through care focuses on providing continuity of care for prisoners with mental health problems. As part of this, no one who is prescribed psychiatric medication should have this discontinued on entry into prison unless a full and formal psychiatric assessment has concluded that this is appropriate. The introduction of the Care Programme Approach is seen as vital to the success of through care, particularly when it comes to planning for aftercare to coincide with a prisoner's release. Access to effective treatments concerns psychological and other non-pharmacological treatments as well as medication (Department of Health, 2001). To tackle suicide and self-harm, the prison service has launched a new policy, which it hopes will lead to changes in the prison environment and staff interventions that are more conducive to prisoner safety (Prison Service, 2001).

The Department of Health and the Prison Service intend to achieve the objectives of the NHS Plan by establishing a programme of mental health in-reach services, starting with prisons identified as having the most pressing needs. Mental health in-reach services will be based on a model of multidisciplinary working in teams similar to those that exist already in the community. The idea is that these teams will ultimately be part of an integrated, modernised mental health service in prison but, to begin with at least, they will focus on prisoners with severe and enduring mental illness. The first phase of in-reach began in 2001/2002. The plan is that, by 2004, 60–70 prisons will have in-reach services (Department of Health, 2001).

The changes described above will be accompanied by a gradual shift in funding responsibility from the Home Office to the NHS. This process began in 2003. Over the next 5 years, prison health will be gradually integrated into the NHS with primary care trusts taking over responsibility for commissioning and providing health care to prisoners. In line with this, annual expenditure on prison health care is set to rise from £90 million to around £136 million.

Substantial changes are being planned to provide much better methods of recording, retrieving and communicating information. This includes developing electronic prison records to improve continuity of care (Department of Health, 2000). These changes will need to be accompanied by information-sharing protocols to safeguard confidentiality. It has been suggested that a nominated key agency could provide a coordinating role so that all aspects of joint working can be considered (Home Office, 1995), although it is not clear yet which body would take on this role.

CONCLUSIONS

Prison health care is the responsibility of numerous professionals who work both within and outside the Prison Service. They deliver care in a highly restrictive environment, and to a population who have disproportionately high levels of ill health, in general, and in terms of mental disorder, in particular.

The modern-day reform of prison health care embraces the concept of multidisciplinary working for prisoners with mental health problems, with secondary mental health care being delivered by mental health in-reach teams adopting the Care Programme Approach. However, because there is no history or culture of multidisciplinary working in prisons, and there is no suggested model for implementation, there is a risk that in-reach services will develop in an *ad-hoc* manner. Just like magistrates court diversion services that have sprung up over the last decade, the end result could be a range of different service models, most of which fail to achieve what they were set up to do (James, 1999).

The disciplined and secure nature of prison can create a number of problems. It may cause high levels of stress among inmates that exacerbate existing mental health problems, and lead to high levels of self-harm or suicide. The dilemma of therapy verses security also arises as a result of attempting to provide for health needs within such a setting.

Front-line staff striving to deliver care within prisons on a daily basis have to overcome the cultural differences, which appear to arise out of a lack of understanding between themselves and their discipline service colleagues with regard to each other's role. These differences may create barriers to effective health care and place those involved under additional pressure.

The past decade has seen the development of various schemes aimed at delivering better health care to prisoners at a local level. In the future, it seems that health care in prisons should be better coordinated and NHS-led. If it is to become a reality, it has to become an integral part of the prison system, involving all those who have day-to-day contact with prisoners for whatever reason.

Interventions designed to address the needs of mentally disordered prisoners have to take into account safeguards that are necessary to protect others from harm. Achieving the right balance requires effective joint working at an agency level. More examples of joint working between agencies involved with mentally disordered offenders, such as multi-agency public protection meetings, are beginning to emerge, but concerns about confidentiality and the needs of the offender being overlooked remain. In order to work effectively, each of the agencies involved needs to develop an understanding of the framework and the ethos in which other agencies work. It is also helpful to have jointly agreed guidelines for sharing information. This is still some way off.

Finally, one of the most controversial issues, but one that cannot be ignored, is that of service user involvement. For those working within secondary mental health services, this is not a new phenomenon but this is a novel concept in a prison setting. Birmingham (1997) commented that little attention has been paid to prisoners' opinions in relation to the development of health care services and, as a consequence service planning, is likely to be one-sided and possibly ineffective. If policy on reforming mental health care emphasises the need to introduce the Care Programme Approach in prisons, this will certainly put the needs and views of the service user firmly into the spotlight and, in doing so, force those involved to confront the very real challenges posed by people who are both patients and prisoners.

References

Birmingham L (1997) Should prisoners have a say in prison health care? British Medical Journal 315: 65–66

Birmingham L (2001) Diversion from custody. Advances in Psychiatric Treatment 7: 198–207

Birmingham L, Mason D, Grubin D (1997) Health screening at first reception into prison. J Forensic Psychiatry 8: 435–439

Dale C and Woods P (2002) Caring for prisoners. Nursing Management 9: 16–21

Department of Health (1990) The Care Programme Approach for people with a mental illness referred to the specialist psychiatric services. London: HMSO

Department of Health (1999) National service framework for mental health—modern standards and service models. London: Department of Health

Department of Health (2000) The NHS plan. A plan for investment a plan for reform. London: HMSO

Department of Health (2001) Changing the outlook: a strategy for developing and modernising mental health services in prisons. London: Department of Health

Department of Health and HM Prison Service (2001) Prison health policy unit and task force annual report 2000–2001. London: Department of Health

Department of Health and Home Office (1992) Review of health and social services for mentally disordered offenders and others requiring similar services. London: HMSO

Droes N S (1994) Correctional nursing practice. Journal of Community Health Nursing 11: 201–210

Fazel S, Danesh J (2000) Serious mental disorder in 23000 prisoners: a systematic review of 62 surveys. Lancet 359: 545–550

Hardy A (1995) Development of the prison medical service, 1774–1895. In: Creese R, Bynum W and Bearn J (eds) The health of prisoners: historical essays. Amsterdam: Clio Medica: 59–80

Harris R (1999) Mental disorder and social order—underlying themes in crime management. In: Webb D and Harris R (eds) Mentally disordered offenders—managing people nobody owns. London: Routledge: 10–26

Health Advisory Committee (1997) The provision of mental healthcare in prisons. London: Home Office

HM Inspectorate of Prisons (1996) Patient or prisoner: a new strategy for healthcare in prisons. London: Home Office

HM Inspectorate of Prisons (1997) Young prisoners: a thematic review by HM Chief Inspector of Prisons for England and Wales. London: Home Office

HM Inspectorate of Prisons (2000) Unjust deserts: a thematic review by HM Chief Inspector of Prisons of the treatment and conditions for unsentenced prisoners in England and Wales. London: Home Office

HM Inspectorate of Prisons (2001) Through the prison gate. London: Home Office

HM Inspectorate of Prisons (2002) Annual report of HM Chief Inspector of Prisons for England and Wales 2002–2003. London: The Stationery Office

HM Prison Service and NHS Executive (1999) The future organisation of prison health care. London: Department of Health

HM Prison Service and NHS Executive (2000) Prison health handbook. London: Department of Health

Home Office (1990) Report on a review by HM Chief Inspector of Prisons: suicide and self-harm in the prison service establishments in England and Wales. London: HMSO

Home Office (1995) Mentally disordered offenders—inter-agency working. London: HMSO

Home Office (1999) The correctional policy framework: protecting the public. London: Home Office

Home Office (2002) Prison population brief, England and Wales: December 2002. London: Home Office

Home Office (2003) The prison population in 2001: a statistical perspective (Findings 195). London: Home Office

James D (1999) Court diversion at 10 years: can it work, does it work and has it a future? Journal of Forensic Psychiatry 10: 507–524

Lart R (1997) Crossing boundaries—accessing community mental health services for prisoners on release. Bristol: Policy Press

Macleod A K, Linehan M M and Williams J M (1992) New developments in the understanding and treatment of suicidal behaviour. Behavioural Psychotherapy 20: 193–218

Mitchison S, Rix K, Renvoize E et al. (1994) Recorded psychiatric morbidity in a large prison for male remanded and sentenced prisoners. Medicine, Science and the Law 34: 324–330

National Probation Service (2002) National Probation Service briefing—an introduction to OaSYS. London: National Probation Service

Parsons S, Walker L and Grubin D (2001) Prevalence of mental disorder in female remand prisons. Journal of Forensic Psychiatry 12: 194–202

Prison Service (1994) Health care standards for prisons in England and Wales. London: Home Office

Prison Service (2000a) Annual report 1999–2000. London: Home Office

Prison Service (2000b) Statutory instruments 1999 No. 728: The prison rules 1999 (as amended by the prison (amendment), rules 2000 and the prison (amendment) (no. 2), rules 2000. London: Home Office

Prison Service (2001) Prevention of suicide and self harm in the Prison Service: an internal review. London: Home Office

Reed J and Lyne M (1997) The quality of health care in prison: results of a year's programme of semi-structured inspections. British Medical Journal 315: 1420–1424

Reed J and Lyne M (2000) Inpatient care of mentally ill people in prison: results of a year's programme of semi-structured inspections. British Medical Journal 320: 1031–1034

Reith M (1988) Community care tragedies. Birmingham: Venture Press

Shakespeare R (2000) A strategy for the management of mentally disordered offenders. Winchester: The Wessex Consortium

Shaw J (2002) NHS National Programme on Forensic Mental Health Research and Development: Prison healthcare. Liverpool: National R & D Programme

Sim J (1990) Medical power in prisons: the Prison Medical Service in England 1774–1989. Milton Keynes: Open University Press

Singleton N, Meltzer H and Gatward R (1998) Psychiatric morbidity among prisoners in England and Wales. London: HMSO

Smith R (1983) The state of the prisons: history of the prison medical services. British Medical Journal 288: 1786–1788

Smith R (1999) Prisoners: an end to second class health care? British Medical Journal 318: 954–955

Smith SS, Baxter VJ and Humphreys MS (2002) The interface between general and prison psychiatry: the consultant's perception. Psychiatric Bulletin 26: 130–132

Tucker R (2001) Nursing in prisons: rising to the challenge. Mental Health Practice 5: 9–11

United Kingdom Central Council for Nursing, Midwifery and Health Visiting (2000) Nursing in secure environments. London: UKCC

Walsh P (1998) What is evidence? A critical review for nursing. Clinical Effectiveness in Nursing 2: 86–93

Webb A (1991) Co-ordination: a problem in public sector management. Policy and Politics 19: 229–241

Chapter **6**

Specific joint working III

Chapter 6A
A forensic mental health liaison scheme: a model of good practice and an evaluation of its multidisciplinary working

Gill Chalder and Nick Griffin

CHAPTER CONTENTS

INTRODUCTION

Health and social care policy in the UK has increasingly emphasised the need for effective multidisciplinary and interagency working (Department of Health, 1989a, 1989b, 1994, 1996; Fried and Rundall, 1994). Many reports have examined the potential benefits of team working, and much of the literature suggests that multidisciplinary team working is the most effective way of providing health and social care (Alexander et al., 1996; Ovretveit, 1997). Some authors have written about the ideal membership of teams but relatively little about the processes that maintain good team functioning.

This section describes one example of effective partnership working between a generic mental health service and specialist forensic mental health provider unit. These services are based approximately 20 miles apart, but have formed a successful multidisciplinary team of clinicians who share the care and management of mentally disordered offenders in a particular community. The findings of a research project, which examined the components of a successful multidisciplinary team working in the scheme, are also described.

Health and social care policy has clearly identified the need to provide appropriate and timely services to mentally disordered offenders.

The 'National service framework for mental health' (Department of Health, 1999a) highlighted the needs of mentally disordered offenders, and described how health care providers in collaboration with the prison service should develop treatment packages and appropriate follow-up. Standards four and five, in particular, highlight the need for those suffering from a severe and enduring mental illness to have access to all services, including secure psychiatric facilities.

The Wolverhampton Forensic Mental Health Services Liaison Scheme was originally established in 1997, following a series of meetings between Wolverhampton Health Authority and managers and clinicians from both provider Trusts. Historically, relationships had been strained. The forensic mental health services in Stafford were commissioning a purpose-built medium-secure unit, and looking to develop innovative and effective ways of working with their neighbouring provider units.

The outcome of these meetings was a genuine desire for both services to work more effectively and rewardingly to the benefit of the patient group and the teams serving their needs, and the development of a joint operational policy for a forensic liaison scheme with defined aims and objectives. Initial funding for a 3-year period was obtained from the Mentally Disordered Offenders Strategic Assistance Fund.

The aims of the scheme were identified as:

- to provide well-informed, effective and rewarding working relationships;
- maximum utilisation of limited resources;
- effective clinical consultation and liaison;
- dissemination of clinical information;
- education and training.

Professionals from the forensic mental health services were allocated sessions to work within the liaison scheme. At the time, this involved a consultant forensic psychiatrist, a consultant forensic clinical psychologist and a senior forensic mental health nurse. The forensic community mental health nurse who operated the existing Court Engagement and Liaison Scheme at the local magistrates court was also included. As the scheme developed, a specialist registrar in forensic psychiatry and a forensic social worker joined the original members. These individuals now belong to a clinical team based at one of the medium-secure units that admit patients from Wolverhampton, the Hatherton Centre in Stafford, thus ensuring continuity and consistency of care.

A senior nurse from the generic mental health services was appointed as local coordinator for the scheme. This was crucial for ensuring that local services remained intimately involved in the scheme, its development and with the relevant patient group. The scheme has developed further and there are now three community mental health nurses, based within local community health teams, acting as scheme coordinators. Each carries a small forensic caseload and is now led by a consultant forensic mental health nurse, providing leadership and expertise.

The composition of this joint general and forensic team would be considered typical of most community mental health teams (Onyett et al.,

1995). The differences are that this liaison team has a specific remit to be involved with mentally disordered offenders, and to support and advise those professionals dealing with them on a daily basis.

One of the core features of this particular liaison scheme is that local services maintain clinical responsibility for the caseload unless transfer of the patient to the secure unit is necessary for a period of time. The model is, therefore, one of 'shared care', with assessment, advice, liaison and support being provided by the team members on any aspects of an individual's management. The care package is coordinated locally and not geographically removed from the individual's area of residence. This ensures that decision-making is not fragmented and assists in effective, regular and clear, unambiguous communication.

Service users from Wolverhampton receive support and intervention from the specialist services, wherever they might be located. This can be in prison, a high-, medium- or low-security hospital, an open psychiatric unit, a bail hostel, police station, in the community or elsewhere. Members of the team travel to conduct assessments wherever the individual may be located at the time of referral to ensure that they remain engaged with services and do not 'slip through the net'. Care is, therefore, coordinated throughout, unmet need can also be identified and appropriate agencies informed of what is required and the rationale behind this.

The specialist forensic mental health team members do not normally provide treatment directly. However, an exception to this is the forensic consultant clinical psychologist, who carries out clinical sessions, in addition to the liaison team meetings and assessments. The main activities of the scheme members as a whole include the following.

- Weekly meetings of the whole team to discuss referrals, arrange assessments, report on active cases, formulate recommendations and conduct individual client reviews.
- Face-to-face assessments in a variety of locations, including the community, bail hostels, rehabilitation hostels, hospital units of all levels of security, the courts and prisons.
- Liaison with various agencies, for example, the police, probation services, social services, housing departments, specialist mental health teams, drug and alcohol teams, and the courts and Crown Prosecution Service, around the cases of individual service users.
- Involvement in the daily Court Engagement and Liaison Scheme at the local magistrates court.
- Liaison with a locally provided Diversion at the Point of Arrest Scheme.
- Clinical supervision by the forensic nurse consultant for the three generic community mental health nurses who carry a forensic caseload.
- Attendance at case conferences, care coordination reviews, multi-agency public protection panel meetings and other relevant clinical meetings.
- Regular practice review meetings, held every 3 months to discuss issues of service development and clinical governance.

- Membership and attendance at various local, regional and national fora concerned with the care and management of mentally disordered offenders.
- Mentoring and shadowing individual professionals to gain an oversight of the working practices of the scheme.
- Dissemination of the model, through Beacon scheme activities and other fora within the West Midlands.

REASONS FOR REFERRAL

There are no specific referral criteria, as the liaison team is reluctant to deter other agencies from referring for advice on a range of issues. In practice, individuals are referred for a variety of reasons, which may include advice on the management of challenging and violent behaviour, assessment of consideration for transfer to a secure environment, advice on risk, for instance, relating to criminal activity, use of weapons, risk to others including children or suicidal behaviour. In addition, there may be the need for consultation on various aspects of the criminal justice system, including the court process, dealing with requests for court reports, how to carry out prison assessments, and information on possible court disposals. A second opinion regarding treatment programmes, accommodation options, relapse prevention, and the level of security required by a particular client may also be an issue for consultation. The benefits of such a scheme to service users has included access to specialist expertise within their own local area. These individuals are known to be difficult to engage at times, so accessibility is critical to ensure they engage and receive appropriate and timely services. Their care package is more robust with appropriate agencies identified and involved. For those placed in medium- or high-secure care, or away from the locality for any other reason, contact is maintained by the forensic liaison team by attendance at case conferences, care coordination reviews, etc. This ensures a smooth pathway when the service user is ready to return to local mental health services. Clinicians from general mental health services report increased confidence and skill in dealing with mentally disordered offenders, knowing that rapid access to support and assistance is available, if required. Service users are less likely to require moving 'out of area' to receive treatment as staff are aware that, if a situation changes and becomes unmanageable, specialist team members will do all they can to assist.

From a commissioner's perspective, pressure on the secure services within the area, both within the National Health Service (NHS) and the private sector, has fallen significantly with the inception of the scheme. Service users placed in the private sector have been repatriated to their area of residence. Regular liaison with the forensic case managers for the West Midlands region ensures that Wolverhampton residents are placed as near to their homes as possible.

In 1998, the scheme successfully applied for 'Beacon status'. This is a Government award for examples of good practice within various categories of health care. Funding was provided to facilitate dissemination of the model, mainly through presentations organised by the team and attendance at academic meetings. This was an excellent and exciting opportunity for team members, both to develop their presentation and liaison skills, and to review their practice with professionals from similar and contrasting services.

It is perhaps ironic that the time and energy devoted to the Beacon Programme detracted from the team's ability to concentrate on the evaluation and further development of the liaison scheme itself. However, the Beacon status did lead to an invitation to apply for the Modernising Government Partnership Awards 2002. As a finalist, the scheme was subject to an external report on its partnership management, which made recommendations that are still being considered as part of the ongoing development programme. There is little doubt that these experiences added significantly to the team's sense of purpose, identity and cohesion.

As part of the liaison scheme's programme of evaluation and development, the team took the opportunity to conduct a research project examining factors contributing to the success of the scheme. All team members met with a team of researchers. A general discussion followed about what the team wanted to achieve and the rationale behind this. Various ideas were debated and it was decided that it would be appropriate to examine in-depth one component of the scheme, namely, how the team itself worked together. This seemed worthwhile in light of the fact that there were circumstances that might make their functioning difficult. These included the geographical distance between the two provider units and the fact that they normally only met together at weekly intervals. Cook et al. (2001) have shown that close proximity between team members increases the opportunity for the passage of information and assists in decision-making. Additionally, for this team, not all individuals were permanent members, which was highlighted by the training role of the specialist registrar in psychiatry, which was a rotational post. Furthermore, at the time that the study was carried out, two members of the team were relatively new to their role within the liaison scheme. This fact may have been reflected in the findings, particularly those aspects that examined role clarity. It was agreed that the research assistant would interview all scheme members.

A qualitative study was carried out which examined team members' perspectives on three aspects of the scheme:

- team working;
- individual membership;
- areas of achievement (and future goals).

A structured interview was undertaken with each participant. Dialogue was then transcribed verbatim and subjected to content analysis. This was done to identify common themes within the team's responses. Nine team members were interviewed, representing 90% of the total scheme membership at that time.

There was a good consensus of opinion within the team regarding what constituted and maintained effective team working. These characteristics were identified as present within the liaison team members.

Examples given included having common aims and objectives, role clarity, respect for each other, and clear and regular communication.

It was felt that this could be improved further by working together more often, although it was recognised that this was not always feasible at the time. The main reasons for this were each team member's commitments outside the liaison scheme varied and that funding was only available for limited sessions. All but one of the forensic team members had only one session allocated to the scheme. Only the clinical psychologist had an extra session allocated for individual therapy time.

It was not that the informal nature of team meetings sometimes detracted from the task in hand, but that this was also deemed vital in maintaining cohesiveness when dealing with what were often perceived as very challenging and complex cases. Several respondents highlighted the positive effect that the team's 'sense of humour' had on overall working relationships. It was also recognised that humour provided an opportunity for resolving conflicts and other issues that might arise.

The study showed a clear understanding of individual member's roles in terms of their own discipline (e.g. psychology or social work) rather than their role within the liaison team. Despite this, everyone seemed clear about how their own role fitted into the group and the work was, therefore, undertaken.

The team generally identified two members as 'leaders', although this role was not stated explicitly within the team structure. Although this did not create problems as such, it did appear to hinder the decision-making process on occasion, if both members were absent from the meeting. Team members recognised that each individual brought unique and valuable skills, knowledge and experience to the scheme. However, difficulty was experienced in trying to elicit training and education needs within the context of the scheme.

In some areas, forensic services have operated in parallel with generic adult mental health services with little integration or 'shared' working practices. The former are often geographically distant from the user's home and involvement with specialist teams has often tended to occur only when crisis point has been reached by local services. The liaison scheme described here has gone a long way to addressing these issues.

This scheme identifies mentally disordered offenders and involves the forensic services at an early stage. Professionals within the local service and a specialist forensic mental health worker conduct joint assessments, visits and treatments. Since the inception of the scheme, communication between local adult mental health services and the specialist forensic mental health service has been greatly enhanced. Furthermore, communication between the four locality-based community mental health teams has also improved. This results in clearer care pathways for mentally disordered offenders, whether they are receiving services from the community mental health teams, inpatient units or are currently placed within the criminal justice system. Communication and liaison has also improved with other agencies, such as the police, Probation Service, courts and prisons, and there is now representation from the scheme on the area's Multi-Agency Public Protection Panel (MAPPS) meetings. Local services have reported feeling more confident when requesting advice, support and, if necessary, an assessment from the specialist forensic mental health service. When a referral to the forensic service is received out of working hours, it is understood that the situation requires an immediate response. This reflects the level of partnership in working and collaboration between the two services. Another obvious advantage is that the team through the liaison scheme itself will often already know the individual. Each team member also has an enhanced knowledge of each other's service limitations, resources, constraints and protocols. The evaluation resulted in a total of nine recommendations for the team to consider and discuss. These mainly centred around more effective working practices, further clarification of roles including leadership and the possibility of an external facilitator at the quarterly practice review meetings.

FUTURE DEVELOPMENTS

With the completion of the Beacon programme, the liaison team members have been able to turn their attention to the future of the scheme. A key feature of the forensic directorate's working philosophy is the application of multiprofessional principles to the strategic and operational management of the service and that team members should lead the development of the model to promote both continuing innovation and consolidation.

The recommendations of the study of the team's multiprofessional working described above, the report on the team's partnership management and the team's own aspirations will be incorporated into a set of strategic objectives and performance measures using a modified balanced scorecard (Robert and David, 1996). This should support both the continuing maturation of the liaison model and of the team itself.

Forensic mental health liaison is a relatively new phenomenon, but one that is rapidly gaining popularity with both commissioners of services and those who are involved in provision of care for mentally disordered offenders. The schemes described here provide just one possible model. Regular practice review meetings have ensured that the team has remained focused, and has the opportunity to modify aims and objectives and consider future developments. This new way of working ensures that service users have readily available access to specialist expertise within their own geographical area. For those who require transfer to a medium secure environment, the same clinical team is responsible for their care, and contact is maintained with local services through the liaison scheme and attendance at care coordination reviews.

Owing to the success of this model, both in clinical and financial terms, the West Midlands regional strategy for forensic mental health services (West Midlands Partnership for Mental Health, 2001) has recommended that all national service framework local implementation teams develop similar schemes by the year 2004. Clinicians involved in this liaison scheme are already in discussion with other local mental health trusts and their commissioners in order to realise this objective.

The evaluation has also demonstrated a high level of job satisfaction, good partnership working and multiagency collaboration. It highlighted an example of effective and rewarding multidisciplinary collaboration involving clinicians from two separate provider units coming together in the same team. All functions of the scheme, ranging from its initial planning, to its performance management and evaluation, were carried out by the team together, and not by individuals or personnel from outside. This served to promote involvement and team cohesiveness, and allowed team members to develop knowledge and skills in areas not previously encountered.

References

Alexander J A, Lichtenstein R, Jinnett K, D'Auno T A and Ullman E (1996) The effects of treatment team diversity and size on assessments of team functioning. Hospital and Health Service Adminstration 41: 37–53

Cook G, Gerrish K and Clarke C (2001) Decision-making in teams: issues arising from two UK evaluations. Journal of Interprofessional Care 15:141–151

Department of Health (1989a) Working for patients. London: HMSO

Department of Health (1989b) Community care in the next decade and beyond. London: HMSO

Department of Health (1994) Working in partnership; a collaborative approach to care. London: HMSO

Department of Health (1996) The health of the nation; building bridges. A guide to arrangements for interagency working for the care and protection of severely mentally ill people. Wetherby: Department of Health

Department of Health (1999a) National service framework—mental health. London: HMSO

Fried B and Rundall T (1994) Groups and teams in health services organisations. In: Shortell S M and Kaluzny A D (eds) Health care management: organisation, design and behaviour, 3rd edn. Albany: Delmar Publishers

Onyett S, Pillinger T and Maijen M (1995) Making community mental health teams work: CMHTs and people who work in them. London: The Sainsbury Centre for Mental Health

Ovretveit J (1997) How to describe interprofessional working. In: Ovretveit J, Mathias P and Thompson T (eds) Interprofessional working for health and social care. London: Macmillan

Robert S K, David P N (1996) Translating strategy into action. The balanced scorecard. Boston, MA: Harvard Business School Press

West Midlands Partnership for Mental Health (2001) Strategy for forensic mental health services (2001–2006). Public Consultation Document. Dudley, West Midlands: Dudley Health Authority

Chapter 6B
Multidisciplinary working in a specialist bail and probation hostel

Jeremy Kenney-Herbert and Jeff Baker

INTRODUCTION

Elliott House, which is located on the outskirts of the suburb of Moseley in Birmingham, United Kingdom, is a specific example of multiagency multidisciplinary working at the interface between the criminal justice and mental health systems. It is an approved bail and probation hostel, now known as approved premises, which specialises in providing a place of residence for mentally disorded offenders. It was established in 1993 as a partnership between the then West Midlands Probation Service and the Regional Forensic Psychiatric Services based at Reaside Clinic, Birmingham.

The impetus for the development of Elliott House arose from within the Probation Service. Probation officers had long recognised that mentally disordered offenders were being remanded in custody for psychiatric reports or other reasons in circumstances where non-mentally disordered offenders charged with similar offences were not. There appeared to be a number of factors associated with this apparent bias. This included lack of understanding and, in many cases, an inappropriate perception of the degree of risk, particularly to others, posed by the defendant and, in some cases, unsuitable housing or no appropriate bail address. It also tended to involve defendants who had lost contact with services, or cases where there were doubts about the ability of the mentally disordered individual to comply with bail and other conditions imposed by courts. At times, inappropriate remands in custody of those clearly suffering from a mental illness arose as a result of concerns about mentally disordered defendants not fully understanding their legal situation, or paradoxically having the ability to participate fully or appropriately in the process. Probation officers recognised that remanding in custody would not be helpful to these individuals' mental health and, in many cases, there appeared to be an unfair and unwarranted loss of liberty, particularly as many such defendants, if convicted, would or could, owing to statutory limitations, ultimately only receive some form of community sentence and would have been unlikely to have been remanded in custody had they not been recognised as mentally disordered. Probation officers had also been concerned about the difficulties they faced in attempting to facilitate re-engagement of the mentally disordered individual brought before the courts with appropriate mental health, social and other services.

As a result of discussion with mental health and criminal justice professionals, planning commenced for the provision of bail accommodation for mentally disordered offenders based in Birmingham. The West Midlands Probation and Forensic Psychiatric Service based in Birmingham then combined to form a partnership to provide the input deemed appropriate using the facility of an existing bail hostel in Edgbaston. After 8 years of consultation, Elliott House bail and probation hostel for mentally disordered offenders opened in 1993.

A senior probation officer manages Elliott House with assistance from another officer as deputy. The probation service officers, known as assistant wardens, ensure that the hostel is staffed at all times by a minimum of two probation service staff. It is subject to the same rules as any other approved probation hostel, including curfew arrangements and particular bail-related conditions, etc. It was opened to cater for 20 male residents and to take referrals from probation officers based in courts or the prisons, rather than other criminal justice or health care professionals, although the latter are not infrequently indirectly involved in the process. The initial aims of Elliott House were to prevent unnecessary remands of mentally disordered offenders in custody and to assist the courts in this respect in making appropriate decisions. As the service developed, Elliott House took on a role, in certain cases, of facilitating the safe reintegration of mentally disordered offenders into the community, including establishing or re-establishing contact between mentally disordered offenders and other services, as appropriate. Although initially designed to take those on bail only, over the years, a large proportion of residents have in fact subsequently been placed at Elliott House as a condition of residence while serving a community rehabilitation order. It has also provided, at times, for a smaller number of individuals on parole licence.

REFERRAL PROCESS AND MULTIDISCIPLINARY MANAGEMENT

The referral process generally includes an initial telephone contact, and initial information gathering according to a purpose-designed protocol, including the faxing or posting of any previous psychiatric reports or assessments that have already been made available to the court or to health professionals within the Prison Service. The decision to accept a referral and then to make a placement available is made by a senior probation officer who may consult with members of the multidisciplinary psychiatric team involved in the work of Elliot House in certain circumstances.

Psychiatric input to Elliot House comes from part of the regional forensic psychiatry service in Birmingham. The multidisciplinary team, led by a consultant forensic psychiatrist, visits the hostel on a regular basis. A forensic community psychiatric nurse provides twice-weekly sessions. An occupational therapist assesses and facilitates group activities within the hostel. Psychological assessment is arranged on an *ad hoc* basis. The involvement of approved social workers, where there is no previous or current social services involvement is also facilitated through the regional forensic psychiatry services. The consultant is supported by junior grade doctors and the work for them, as well as students and trainees from other clinical backgrounds, is considered an extremely valuable and, in many ways, unique learning and educational opportunity. A local general practitioner provides primary care services for residents. For those with existing contacts with mental health services or previous contacts, every attempt is made to continue involvement from those services where practical. However, as the service at Elliott House receives national referrals, this is not always feasible.

Once a referral has been accepted and the future resident has arrived at the hostel, there is an induction programme, which a member of hostel staff takes them through. The rules and regulations of the hostel are explained and appropriate written information is provided. As a condition of an offer of a place, all residents need to have agreed to the placement at Elliott House. It is explained to them that they will be assessed by members of the multidisciplinary forensic psychiatric team, and that some information may be shared between the mental health care team and members of the hostel staff in order to enhance the individual care and appropriate management of each resident, and to promote their health and safety, and also that of others around them. Hostel staff establish what medication residents have previously been prescribed and make arrangements for this to be continued until the psychiatric team assesses them.

The forensic psychiatric team aims to assess new admissions to Elliott House within 72 hours. This initial contact is generally with the forensic community psychiatric nurse or a medical member of the team. It is intended, at first, to provide an overview of the individual's psychiatric history and current mental state, as well as any treatment and potential management difficulties, including those that might arise out of concerns over real or potential risks of self-harm or harm to others. It is made clear again at this stage to residents that some information may need to be shared and discussed with probation staff, and the reasons behind this. Where treatment is being provided through an existing contact with mental health services, this is continued where possible, and appropriate contact made with the local team informing them of the patient's placement at the hostel. Where it is apparent that treatment needs to be adjusted or changed, this will be discussed and implemented, particularly if there is no pre-existing treatment plan. In a majority of cases, it is found to be appropriate for further assessment and follow-up to continue with mental health care team members, as it were on an 'out patient' basis with the bailee or probationer staying as a resident at Elliot House for a period of time, and probation staff providing day-to-day care and management and specialist liaison.

The multidisciplinary nature of working at Elliot House can be exemplified by the way in which the decision to return a bailee to the court is made between hostel probation staff and the visiting forensic team. The decision to breach is ultimately a matter for the Probation Service; however, where the individual's unstable mental state is a contributing factor in their conditions of bail being broken, or when there is a lack of clarity to the role of their mental state and their behaviour, the decision to breach would also involve members of the forensic psychiatric team. This allows the potential for a change in the management plan, which may curtail future offending behaviour or behaviour that leads to the person being in breach of their conditions of residence. Occasionally, breach proceedings can be prevented, so long as the resident's behaviour is not felt to pose a danger to the local community, where alternative strategies may be utilised by hostel staff, as recommended by the forensic team. Additionally, members of the forensic team may take a more realistic and longer-term view than hostel staff, by arguing that an increasingly stable mental state of an individual would correspondingly result in a reduction of offending behaviour over time.

THE REVIEW PROCESS

The cornerstone of interagency multidisciplinary working at Elliott House is the weekly review meeting. Residents are assessed and reviewed by medical and nursing members of the multidisciplinary psychiatric team. Following this clinic, a senior probation officer, probation hostel staff and psychiatric team members, including psychiatrists, the occupational therapist and community psychiatric nurse (CPN) meet to review all current residents. The various aspects of the individual's legal, social housing and psychiatric status are discussed. Probation and hostel staff are able to provide a description and overview of the resident's presentation during the preceding week, and raise any concerns or other issues. This and any additional information is often invaluable in informing the mental health care professionals of issues relating to mental state that may not have been apparent during formal assessment. The mental health care staff will generally review the psychiatric history, the resident's current mental state and, particularly, raise matters relating to the individuals' potential risk to themselves or others. Clinical treatment and management plans will be explained and elaborated with the potential role of the probation and hostel staff in this context being discussed and agreed. Risk assessment and management plans are developed and formal minutes of the meetings are recorded. This forum often generates lively discussion around the roles and different perceptions of each agency's functions, responsibilities and ethical and professional frameworks and, with time, has led to enhanced care and understanding of the needs of mentally disordered individuals bailed to or on probation at Elliot House.

The discussions frequently lead to liaison with solicitors and other probation officers as well as agencies, such as housing or social services, in relation to the future management of a particular resident. On occasions, residents may have raised sensitive issues either with hostel staff or with mental health professionals. Careful consideration is given to how such information is used and conveyed to others in discussion with the resident in question, and it is always made clear that all information discussed at the meeting is confidential. Where issues that relate to the potential for risks to others are raised and thought to be of such significance that action may have to be taken, attempts are made to involve the individual concerned in discussions of what might need to happen as a result of the risks identified. In such circumstances, it is common for one of the senior probation officers and consultant psychiatrist to meet jointly with the individual resident in an attempt to gain their agreement to take action and, if appropriate, facilitate the sharing of information with other individuals or agencies as necessary. This element of the meeting is crucial, as probation staff, in partnership with the forensic team, can have a united approach to involving local and more distant services from initial contact with a resident, devising care packages, through to returning the individual back to their local area, with the necessary professional and personal relationships in place.

Probation and hostel staff, as well as the occupational therapist in the area of skills relating to independent living, educational background and constructive activity, assess residents. Weekly sessions, including assertiveness training, fitness, mental health awareness, drugs awareness and education are available, the latter involving both in-house and external agencies. The hostel has a small physical training area with equipment. Use is also made of a nearby occupational therapy day facility and some residents are encouraged to become involved in voluntary work.

STUDY EVALUATION

The characteristics of residents at Elliott House between August 1994 and April 1996 were described by Geelan et al. (1998). During this period, the vast majority were bailees. At that time, fewer than 10% were on probation orders, a figure which has steadily risen to the current time when more than one in three residents is on a probation order at any one time. Over half are of no fixed abode and 74% have had previous contact with psychiatric services both as inpatients and outpatients. One-third were in contact with mental health services at the time of arrest and approximately 40% had a history of deliberate self-harm. Over half the residents had a diagnosis of a primary psychotic disorder, such as schizophrenia, and a further 10% had a major affective disorder. High rates of drug and alcohol misuse and dependence were identified. Approximately 20% were diagnosed with a personality disorder and around 5% were diagnosed as suffering from a learning disability or some other form of psychiatric disorder. A significant minority were found to suffer from no disorder, as such, and had been charged or convicted of a range of offences. More than one-third involved violence and approximately one-third were property related. A significant minority, approximately 5%, had been charged with or convicted of sexual offences. In a majority of cases, those charged with offences involving supplying illicit substances are excluded from the hostel on the basis of the potential problems that might arise from such activity within the facility.

Potential outcomes for residents convicted of offences include probation or community rehabilitation orders, with a condition of residence at Elliott House, or as directed by the probation officer. There may also be conditions of psychiatric treatment attached. Some residents are referred to hospital for inpatient admission and may return to the hostel at the end of that time. Other residents may receive alternative forms of non-custodial sentences, such as conditional discharge or community punishment order. Some are sentenced to imprisonment. A study of 21 residents of Elliot House made subject to community rehabilitation orders with a requirement for psychiatric treatment, described by Clark et al. (2002), showed that most of these individuals had a diagnosis of schizophrenia and a low rate of reoffending whilst at the hostel. Unfortunately, long-term data about reoffending and subsequent contact with mental health care services for those subject to a community rehabilitation order with conditions of psychiatric treatment are not available (Clark et al., 2002).

CONCLUSION

Interagency and multidisciplinary working with mentally disordered offenders clearly has advantages, and has been discussed widely and proposed and promoted as an ideal repeatedly over time and by many (Department of Health and Home Office, 1992). Most mentally disordered offenders have multiple complex needs and pose a considerable challenge. There are frequent misperceptions and misunderstandings between criminal justice and mental health service providers in relation to the potential roles and responsibilities, and indeed powers, of each agency in such cases. Challenging these can bring about conflict and unhelpful interactions, but these differences can only be explored and resolved, and the care of those involved thus improved, with commitment and a willingness to listen and learn on both sides. Clear understanding between criminal justice and mental health agencies not only dispels such misperceptions, but also can increase the opportunities for collaborative and complementary working to deal with complex problems. For example, in the area of assessing potential risk to others, the National Probation Service and psychiatric services may have different approaches, but there will be some overlap. These approaches can, therefore, be summative and together help to reach a more comprehensive risk management plan, which may involve resources that would only otherwise have been available to one agency. In circumstances where offending behaviour or risk to others is predominantly related to mental health issues, psychiatric treatment and future care will be the major consideration. In some cases, the relationship between mental health problems and offending behaviour is not clear and, in some, the two may be unrelated. In such circumstances, the role of criminal justice agencies, such as the National Probation Service, may need to be more prominent.

There clearly is an important educational role for professionals from each of the fields of mental health and probation in relation to one another, and the ability, through joint working, to grasp and understand the role of others, as well as gain knowledge in areas outside their own expertise. There is, of course, a constant potential tension between the approaches of each agency. Although the probation service originally rose out of a social work-based ethos, in more recent years there has been a deliberate re-emphasis upon public protection driven by Government policy. This is evident in the marked contrast between pre-sentence reports in the past, which were very much of a social work-related nature, with a comprehensive background history and information, compared to those produced now, which are structured around risk assessment and management, and with less overt reference to the welfare of the offender. Psychiatric team members have their own professional and ethical frameworks within which to perform their clinical duties. Their emphasis will be on the health and well-being of the individual resident or patient, although there is always a need to be aware of the interests of others in society in relation to potential risk from the individual in the care of mentally disordered offenders. It has been the experience of those working at Elliott House that, when such tensions arise and specific issues are discussed openly, and in a clear detailed way, a practical and sensible way of moving forward can usually be found.

Elliott House has succeeded in meeting evident unmet need for some mentally disordered offenders. It has prevented many unnecessary remands in custody and enabled the mental health requirements of mentally disordered offenders to be addressed. It has been a successful partnership between one criminal justice agency and mental health services. It has overcome philosophical and procedural differences between these agencies through open and frank discussion and agreements on roles and responsibilities. It represents a modern approach of working with mentally disordered offenders that could and should be replicated in other areas of the criminal justice system.

References

Clark T, Kenney-Herbert J, Baker G and Humphreys M (2002) Psychiatric probation orders: failed provision or future panacea? Medicine, Science and the Law 42: 58–63

Department of Health and Home Office (1992) Review of health and social services for mentally disordered offenders and others requiring similar services (The Reed Report). London: HMSO

Geelan S, Griffin N and Briscoe J (1998) A profile of residents at Elliot House, the first approved bail and probation hostel specifically for mentally disordered offenders. Health Trends 30: 101–105

Chapter 6C
Multidisciplinary statutory follow-up of conditionally discharged patients

Sharon Riordan

This section is based on research that looked at the statutory community follow-up of those conditionally discharged restricted hospital order patients being actively supervised in the West Midlands at 1 April 2000 (Riordan et al., 2000a, 2000b, 2004). The disciplines of medicine, nursing and social services were represented in the responses given regarding the benefits and deficits of multidisciplinary statutory community supervision.

INTRODUCTION

Research has shown that restricted hospital order patients are a distinct group with very complex needs (Street, 1998). The restricted patient population, although not homogeneous, mainly consists of single unemployed men suffering from severe mental illness, namely schizophrenia, with an extensive history of prior contact with psychiatric services, a history of non-compliance with treatment and comorbid substance misuse, often further complicated by episodes of self-harm. They have committed a grave offence and, collectively, they have an extensive record of criminality and early onset of offending (Riordan et al., 2002a). As a group, they represent the patients at the core of forensic mental health care, both as inpatients and subsequently in the community after conditional discharge has been sanctioned.

The benefit of conditional discharge was recognised as far back as 30 years ago (Walker and McCabe, 1973). Conditionally discharged patients were matched one-for-one with controls from amongst those hospital order patients who had no apparent arrangements for aftercare. There were 22 pairs. Of those that received planned aftercare, only four had been reconvicted during the follow-up period compared with 13 of those who had received no aftercare. The authors were able to show an association between aftercare and favourable outcomes, and concluded that their data provided a strong case for intensifying efforts to provide this, particularly for high-risk groups.

More recent research examined the Home Office files of all those patients conditionally discharged from hospital between 1987 and 1990 (Street, 1998). Seventy per cent had a criminal record when the restriction order was imposed. Of these, 61% had previously been convicted of a sexual or violent offence. The study highlighted a number of factors that suggest some value in the use of restricted hospital orders, namely low rates of reconviction and the ability of professionals to share responsibility in the management of potentially dangerous mentally disordered offenders.

In a detailed study, the supervision of restricted patients was examined from a wide variety of perspectives (Dell and Grounds, 1995). Responsible medical officers, social supervisors and patients considered supervision valuable. In particular, individuals found that social supervisors gave assistance in numerous ways, including help with housing, benefits, and moral and human support. The patients themselves found that conditional discharge was a welcome guarantee that they could get treatment and a hospital bed if they required it. However, factors such as frequent staff changes compromised the effectiveness of the supervision process. One in four of the sample was recalled at some point in time but, in 40% of the cases, the issue of public protection was not a consideration.

What is apparent from all of the studies is that the process of statutory community aftercare for conditionally discharged patients is by and large successful. What has not been addressed in any detail is why this should be the case. It could be that the legal constraint forces both patients and clinicians to engage with one another and comply with Home Office requirements and regulations. It might also be that legal enforcement provides the framework within which patients, professionals and carers have the opportunity to form good relationships with each other, allowing successful supervision.

By the time individuals are considered for conditional discharge, they may have spent a considerable period of time in a structured, therapeutic and often secure environment. At the point of conditional discharge, the work done by the multidisciplinary team to control and reduce the risk is measured and considered. In a majority of cases, restricted patients will have had some unescorted leave from the hospital and, in some cases, they will be essentially living away from the hospital when the conditional discharge is sanctioned.

An order for conditional discharge may specify a number of requirements considered appropriate for the welfare of the patient and for the protection of the public. These might include place of residence, and that the patient may not visit a particular area or contact specific individuals. The patient has a designated social supervisor, most frequently a social worker, but occasionally a probation officer or community psychiatric nurse (Home Office, 1997). A psychiatrist is identified to act as responsible medical officer (RMO; Home Office, 1987). Both the RMO and social supervisor have statutory duties and responsibilities in relation to the care and follow-up of the conditionally discharged restricted hospital order patient, and the philosophy of a close team membership means that disciplines from all agencies involved in the patient care work as an integrated team and all relevant information concerning a patient is shared amongst those involved in the patient's care. Forensic community psychiatric nurses are fully integrated in the team, and take an active role in the discharge and community aftercare of the patients. The purpose of supervision is to monitor the patient's mental state continually, to maintain their mental health, to offer social support, to assess the level of risk the patient poses to themselves or others at any particular time, and aid in the protection of the public by facilitating the patient's return to the community.

MULTIDISCIPLINARY PERCEPTIONS OF STATUTORY COMMUNITY AFTERCARE

Good things about supervision

Legal framework

The consensus of opinion across all of the professional groups interviewed is that the main benefit of conditional discharge is the legal framework. Professionals expressed the belief that statutory provision ensured continued engagement with psychiatric services for patients, leading to enhanced compliance with treatment and follow-up. The legal framework provides structure and boundaries, particularly for those with a previous history of difficult behaviour. The legal framework was also seen as a way of minimising risk to the individual and the general public, and as supporting the professional relationship between the team, the patient and their families. Many thought that, without statutory supervision, their patients would be lost to follow-up. In addition, professionals thought prolonged and intensive supervision was effective in enhancing patient insight into their illness, leading to greater patient independence.

> Without the framework he would be lost to services . . . without conditional discharge he would have gone off the rails a long time ago. He has a vast history of drug abuse and criminality so therefore the legal framework has given him boundaries. Having the lever of control helps us to keep him well in the community.

Compliance

Many patients had a history of non-compliance with medication and subsequent disengagement with services. In the case of one man with mental illness, the intensive follow-up and the close professional relationship that had developed between the patient and nurse, were instrumental factors in the patient being able to verbalise his distress, and enabled the CPN to pick up signs of relapse early, thus avoiding hospitalisation, or at least reducing the length of hospital stay for those patients who were admitted.

> Because he had such close contact with the service, on two occasions he was unwell and felt able to get help quickly. Things were dealt with quickly and that was positive for him and the service. It avoided a long readmission and on the second occasion it avoided readmission altogether.

Risk   Comments about the benefit of supervision from the point of view of risk reduction featured commonly in the responses. The degree of control over where the patient lived, the intensive multidisciplinary supervision and the use of compulsory drug screening were seen as helpful.

> His offence was drug related in part and after conditional discharge he started to smoke cannabis. The restriction order assisted us in giving him regular urine screening. It helps minimise the risk.

Repeated interagency collaboration between the psychiatric services, the police and social services was considered a benefit of statutory supervision, and an important aspect in reducing potential risk of harm to others. Also, the close monitoring of patients allows for the early detection of relapse and the ability to take prompt action when any problems manifest. Many professionals felt that, without supervision, patients would reoffend. One social supervisor commented:

> Without supervision I'd be very worried about him reoffending. In fact I'd almost guarantee it. The reason for that is he wouldn't comply with medication, he'd abuse drugs, get into a financial crisis, he'd exploit others and that would lead to an offence.

Relationships   The legal framework was said to enhance multidisciplinary team, patient and family inter-relationships, where the assistance and support of the family were perceived as key factors of successful supervision. There were many comments about the positive impact that working with conditionally discharged patients for a substantial length of time prior to conditional discharge had on the therapeutic relationship. A number of social supervisors working in medium-secure settings mentioned the value of this in particular. The development of close relationships between social supervisors and the patients' families was made clear in a number of cases.

> His close family are very positive regarding the restriction order. This has helped having had time to build these relationships in the medium secure unit. These relationships are very helpful.

The continuity of care was seen as very beneficial, where families and carers were said to be able to provide the clinical team with vital information, and express concerns they have about the patient, assisting the development of proactive rather than reactive care, thereby avoiding crisis situations.

> I can liaise with his parents and carers and get good feedback . . . I have a good relationship with his family, they are an alliance to the team.

Bad things about supervision

Legal framework   Although the legal framework was identified as a major factor in successful statutory supervision, paradoxically the legal framework was mentioned most commonly as a negative feature of supervision. Supervision was, in the main, seen to last too long, encouraging patients' dependency on psychiatric services and, in some cases, causing damage to the therapeutic relationship. Social supervisors, in particular, disliked the control aspect of their role, which they considered caused conflict in some cases.

> It puts you in the role of a social policeman. With a conditional discharge you are acting as an agent of the Home Office. The patient sees you as a grass to the RMO for failing to take medication, breaking the conditions of the conditional discharge, etc.

Drug misuse   Nurses raised the problems caused by patients who abused drugs in the community on a number of occasions, although one nurse commented that compulsory drug testing, which had been imposed on a number of patients, had compromised the therapeutic relationship and damaged the supervision process.

RECOMMENDATIONS FOR CHANGE

Accommodation

There were a number of observations about the difficulties faced in obtaining appropriate accommodation for conditionally discharged patients. It was felt that patients would, in some cases, benefit from being geographically closer to their families for additional support. A need for access to more supported housing, particularly for the more vulnerable patients, who were subject to exploitation from various sectors of society, was voiced, whilst other professionals recognised that some patients should have more independent accommodation in order to reduce the stigma associated with living in a mental health hostel in the community. Nurses, social supervisors and consultant psychiatrists highlighted the need for a change of accommodation in some cases for their patients, owing to the high level of illicit drug use in the area where they lived. One nurse described very clearly the implications of vulnerable patients living in such areas.

> We had to move him to another area because of his drug problems. He's abused by drug dealers.

One supervisor felt that one patient would benefit from a change of accommodation owing to his ethnicity, whilst others recognised that some individuals were suffering from the negative effects of the stigma of being an offender patient in the community. Therefore, specialist services with the confidence to be involved in housing offender patients were also suggested.

> He doesn't feel that there are enough people from his ethnic background in his area . . . he feels out on a limb.

Staffing issues

In response to the significant levels of black people in secure psychiatric environments and in restricted hospital order populations, in particular, there was an acknowledgment for the need to employ more black staff on clinical teams from all professions. Nurses, in particular felt that there should be more staff from ethnic minority groups to undertake nursing responsibilities for those under statutory supervision. In two cases, there was evidence that nurses had experienced difficulties in their relationships with their patient's families in this respect.

I'm a white woman, not exactly accepted by the family but tolerated. The patient himself doesn't have a problem with me.

Drug misuse

There were responses from representatives of all professions identifying a need for more effective means of drug misuse prevention. Social supervisors and psychiatrists thought that standardising drug and alcohol testing would be useful, particularly if drug or alcohol misuse had been a significant factor in terms of relapse.

Transfer of care

A number of professionals from nursing and social work thought it would be beneficial for their patients to be transferred to the care of a local community mental health team. One supervisor felt that the specialist forensic team was keeping patients in their care too long, creating problems for both patients and services. Some comments made by nursing staff indicated that they felt that the attitudes of those working in general psychiatry towards forensic patients had changed over recent times.

Now that local services have seen what we do in the medium secure unit and our continuity of care, etc. this has helped to improve our relations with local services.

DISCUSSION

Professionals in forensic services recognise the value of the involvement of various different members of the multidisciplinary clinical team and family support in the conditional discharge process. Furthermore, the support of carers by the team and the requirement of professionals to respond to the needs of people from a variety of ethnic and cultural backgrounds are given a high priority (Riordan et al., 2002b). In forensic mental health care, the important elements in effective supervision are the development of a close working relationship with the patient, their family and the maintenance of a good liaison between team members. Teamwork and close communication have previously been highlighted as key factors in any work with offender patients (Prins, 1983).

All those involved in the process agree that statutory community aftercare is an effective process for assisting in the maintenance of good mental health for restricted patients, and for minimising the risk of harm to themselves and the public. It allows for the development of good relationships between patients, carers and professionals, enhances patient insight into their mental illness, and reduces the chance of the patient disengaging from psychiatric services.

On the basis of the opinions expressed here, it may be tempting to suggest that the long-established process of conditional discharge might, in some ways, be viewed as a template for a model of psychiatric community aftercare, for a substantial group of patients, their carers and clinical teams, that is successful from a wide variety of different perspectives. This would be an oversimplistic way of interpreting the findings of the research. Whilst there does seem to be some inherent property of the process of conditional discharge that is likely to have to do with a relatively prolonged period of contact with inpatient treatment services, careful, steady preparation and rehabilitation towards a particular package of community aftercare, with a commitment from specific named individuals, in the form of the social supervisor and responsible medical officer, to that package of care, and access to appropriate accommodation and other forms of support, and then the detailed scrutiny of the Mental Health Review Tribunal in restricted cases, the limits associated with the requirements of the legislation are only one small part of the equation. Perhaps most important is the fact that mental health legislation imposes responsibilities upon both the patient and the clinical team, which inevitably leads to the need for intensive, individually tailored, and expertly monitored and delivered forms of treatment and management, which in turn require appropriate resourcing. Without this and the expertise developed within specialist services, the process, and the opinions of those involved in it, despite the presence of an externally imposed legislative framework, would be likely to be very different.

References

Dell S and Grounds A T (1995) The discharge and supervision of restricted patients. London: HMSO

Home Office (1987) Mental Health Act 1983: supervision and after-care of conditionally discharged restricted patients notes for the guidance of supervising psychiatrists. London: Home Office and Social Security

Home Office (1997) Notes for the guidance of social supervisors Mental Health Act 1983: supervision and after-care of conditionally discharged restricted patients. London: Home Office, Department of Health and Welsh Office

Prins H (1983) The care of the psychiatric prisoner— discharge into the community and its implications. Medicine, Science and the Law 23: 79–86

Riordan S, Smith H and Humphreys M (2002a) Conditionally discharged restricted patients and the need for long-term medium security. Medicine, Science and the Law 42: 339–343

Riordan S, Smith H and Humphreys M (2002b) Alternative perceptions of statutory community aftercare: patient and responsible medical officer views. Journal of Mental Health Law No 7:119–129

Riordan S, Donaldson S and Humphreys M (2004) The imposition of restricted hospital orders: potential effects of ethnic origin. The International Journal of Law and Psychiatry 27: 171–177

Street R (1998) The restricted hospital order: from court to the community (Research Study 186). London: HMSO

Walker N and McCabe S (1973) Crime and insanity in England, Vol. 2. Edinburgh: Edinburgh University Press

Further reading

Cope R and Ndegwa D (1991) Ethnic differences in admission to a regional secure unit. Journal of Forensic Psychiatry 1: 365–378

Dolan M, Coorey P and Kulupana S (1993) An audit of recalls to a special hospital. Journal of Forensic Psychiatry 4: 249–260

Howat J G M and Kontny E L (1982) The outcome for discharged Nottingham long-stay in-patients. British Journal of Psychiatry 141: 590–594

Humphreys M, Kenney-Herbert J and Gray C (1998) Restricted hospital orders; a survey of forensic psychiatrists' practice and attitudes to their use. Journal of Forensic Psychiatry 9: 245–247

Chapter **7**

Multidisciplinary aspects of the Care Programme Approach

Aidan Houlders

INTRODUCTION

The concept and practice of multidisciplinary team working in health care overall, and as a vehicle for the delivery of mental health care services, in particular, is not new. It has developed as part of the evolution of services in response to the realisation that people with mental health problems typically have a variety of health and social care needs that cannot be effectively managed by one discipline or practitioner alone. The importance attached to multidisciplinary working may be seen in the number of Government mental health service publications that have stated very clearly the need for a collaborative approach both within and between service purchasers and providers (Department of Health, 1995a).

The Care Programme Approach (CPA) is a relatively new development in the English system of delivering mental health care services and was introduced in 1991 (Department of Health, 1990). In a policy booklet, the Government stated that the CPA is *the* framework in the delivery of mental health care services, and made reference throughout to the importance of multidisciplinary working in the delivery of mental health care services to patients and stated that this should be initiated at the very first point of contact with a patient (Social Services Inspectorate and National Health Service (NHS) Executive, 1999).

This chapter aims to explore, how a 'forensic' Care Programme Approach differs from the CPA provided in general adult care psychiatric

[handwritten margin note: Forensic, Criminal Justice sys., Home Office]

services. In forensic practice, there is a need to recognise that patients may experience certain 'advantages' and 'disadvantages', which relate to their position in the process of the criminal justice system or their relationship with other bodies, such as the Mental Health Unit of the Home Office. There are a number of factors, operating in and outside the medium-secure facility, which affect the delivery of a forensic mental health care service. These factors are broadly dealt with in the examination of the organisation's approach to the delivery of that service, and how its policies and procedures impact on the practices of a forensic multidisciplinary team.

THE CARE PROGRAMME APPROACH

General comment

At Section 117, the Mental Health Act 1983 places a duty on health and social services to provide aftercare for patients who had been compulsorily detained under Sections 3, 37, 45A, 47 and 48. Section 117 discharge planning meetings take place at the end of the inpatient period to finalise arrangements for a patient's follow-up. The nature of this planning has tended to be somewhat idiosyncratic and, at times, rather arbitrary. All other patients can be discharged without formal planning of their aftercare arrangements, although the principles of good practice should dictate otherwise.

The CPA was introduced in response to public concern about the aftercare and supervision of people with mental health problems living in the community. It had become clear that so-called 'care in the community', as a response to the hospital closure plan was not working properly (Ministry of Health, 1962). A disturbing situation emerged where mental health patients were being discharged without proper arrangements being made for their follow-up in the community. A number of mental health inquiries reported on the apparent failures in the systems of care (see Sheppard, 1996; Reith, 1998).

The Social Services Inspectorate team in 1995 reported on its findings about the implementation of the CPA, which they concluded was patchy across the country (Department of Health, 1995b). They also noted that the CPA was commonly implemented at the discretion of the responsible medical officer (RMO) at the point of a patient's discharge. It was further observed that workers in health and social care appeared to be duplicating the processes of assessment under the CPA and Care Management (NHS Community Care Act 1990; see Bailey, 2000).

The Government produced a number of booklets '. . . to encourage mental health service providers and practitioners to apply the CPA framework to any individual in contact with the psychiatric service at *any* stage, not purely at the point of discharge. . . .' (Department of Health, 1996). Multidisciplinary working was seen as the main vehicle for the assessment, planning, organising, delivering and monitoring of services. 'Effective care coordination in mental health services—modernising the Care Programme Approach' builds on related government initiatives, such as the 'Mental Health Service national service framework'(Department of Health, 1999a), which sets out to modernise delivery of mental health care services through partnership and integration of health and social care agencies. The CPA '… is *the* framework for care coordination and resource allocation in mental health care …' (Department of Health, 1990). The revised CPA addresses matters that have concerned mental health care practitioners for some time. It outlines changes described in 'The Care Programme Approach Association' booklet (CPA Association, 2001). This provides some guidance on the CPA, covering all the main elements, with particular reference to the role of the care coordinator. Of special note in terms of multidisciplinary team working in forensic mental health services is the expectation that the CPA will be integrated for assessment purposes with care management (NHS and Community Care Act, 1990) and that assessment procedures will be a single activity applied at the *first* point of contact regardless of setting, including for instance the high-secure psychiatric hospitals or prisons. The revised CPA also restates the importance of support for carers, and for their needs to be separately assessed under the provisions of the Carer (Recognition and Services) Act 1995 (Department of Health, 2003). There is an expectation that providers will undertake an audit of their CPA programmes and there is centrally generated guidance on how this should be undertaken (Department of Health, 1996).

The CPA then has become the framework for the delivery of mental health services, and should also be used at the first point of contact in relation to all users, regardless of where they are. It should also include those individuals first identified, or already known to services, who are within the Prison System. The spirit of the policy appears to be about delivery of integrated mental health care services through the proper process of comprehensive social and health care assessment, gaining an understanding of the needs of patients and their carers, and providing consistent, systematic and well-coordinated care and management service through joint health and social planning, which is subject to regular review and audit. In this way, it may be said to be, as it were, a blueprint for multidisciplinary and multiagency working.

THE CARE PROGRAMME APPROACH IN FORENSIC MENTAL HEALTH SERVICES

One approach used when the CPA was introduced in 1991 was to create a person-centred computerised system of storing and retrieving patient information. The care plan template can then be completed and regularly updated by a clinical team for each of its patients. The plan is available for inspection by authorised staff, if they need to refer to it for guidance in the absence of clinicians who are directly responsible for the patient's care, for example, responding to a situation concerning a patient as part of an 'out-of-hours' service.

In addition to the basic personal information, there can be other sections in the document, which detail the patient's psychiatric history, including any previous contacts with the forensic mental health care service and/or the criminal justice system. This information provides the background that sets the context for the circumstances leading up to the patient's admission into a secure psychiatric setting. Other sections deal with the assessment of risk and its management, early warning signs of relapse and actions to be taken in the event of a deterioration of the patient's mental state. This information may be found in other CPA documentation used in other mental health care services. However, the various sections and the computerised form of the recording allow for a full description of the patient's past and current situation. The design of the form avoids the 'tick box' approach to recording information. Particular attention can be paid to the risk factors and any issues that relate to victim perspectives.

Using this model where it is appropriate, each member of the clinical team is expected to provide information, which is then written into the care plan under the relevant section, that is, planned activities as part of the patients' follow-up when they are discharged, etc.

The document would normally be compiled together with the patient and his carers. One section does allow for the recording of disagreements between the patient and his clinical team. One of the final sections sets out *measures of success*. These can include such things as 'need for readmission', 'avoidance of alcohol or illicit substance misuse', 'gaining employment/training courses', etc. These measures of success are related to the *objectives* of the team and patient, which form another section of the care plan.

This document frequently contains sensitive information, which the patient may find difficult to accept, especially when it deals with the circumstances leading up to his admission. It is important, therefore, that the recorded information is factually correct and accurately reports the opinions of team members and the patient because, as stated elsewhere, the document may be shared with other colleagues outside the forensic service.

The CPA in forensic mental health care concentrates on patients' clinical needs as well as offending behaviours or behaviours that might put them at risk of serious harm to themselves and/or others. The care plan is the heart of this process, and is a document that should be constructed in a partnership between the patient and the clinical team, which will take into account the views of others, for example, patient's carers/family, victim perspective and any additional information required by other agencies to facilitate the objectives of the care plan. The crafting of the care plan, which is a prerequisite to service delivery, must take account of the risks posed by patients. It is a confidential document but is made in the knowledge that other workers outside the forensic setting may have access to it in order to realise its objectives, especially as they relate to progression of an individual into community living. The care plan, which is made through a process of joint agreement and in consultation with the patient, becomes a document to share with carers, other workers in the mental health care system and, where required, representatives of other agencies, for example, those involved in the criminal justice system and community-based services, such as accommodation providers.

The Government, through the Home Office, directs that an offender's treatment and rehabilitation plan, where it relates to arrangements allowing access to the public, must take into account the *victim perspective*, and gain the views, where possible, of the victim or the victim's family. The National Probation Service and one of its victim support units usually deal with these matters. Multi-Agency Protection Panels (MAPPs) have also been created to consider the position and protection of the public, as well as victims and/or their families in response to patients returning to live in the community. This aspect of care planning is not dealt with overtly in the policy booklet on the CPA but forms a major part of the planning of offender patient's care in a forensic service.

Patients may be subjected to restrictions imposed by the Home Office and/or the criminal justice system, which will primarily be concerned with public protection issues. The views of health and social care practitioner assessments on the risks a patient actually poses are required before a decision is made to give ministerial consent. Providing a care plan in a forensic mental health care service is, therefore, not simply about managing the internal organisation of a health care setting. It is also about demonstrating to a sceptical audience the process of rehabilitation, and community-based arrangements, providing levels of support and care, which ensure a patient's safety, and the protection of the public. The care plan should instil a confidence in all interested parties that it is safe to work with patients in a non-secure community-based setting.

It is interesting to note that, even if there is a robust care plan that caters for the specific needs of victims or their families and where there may be multiagency agreement on the plan to go ahead with a community-based placement, the whole thing can be swept aside following adverse publicity or media attention. This is another matter, which does not feature in the CPA policy document, but it is a real issue for forensic multidisciplinary teams, as they attempt to provide an effective and safe aftercare service. How these additional dimensions are managed, rests with the health care provider's organisational policies, its procedures and its multidisciplinary team.

ORGANISATIONAL ASPECTS OF MULTIDISCIPLINARY TEAM WORKING IN A FORENSIC MENTAL HEALTH SETTING

This chapter will describe one particular form of clinical team approach to multidisciplinary working. However, this is not something that can take place in isolation but is linked to other practices that are also multidisciplinary activities, and form part of the internal organisation and management of this particular forensic mental health service.

A clinical team may be composed of the following practitioners:

- a consultant forensic psychiatrist;
- a specialist registrar;
- a registrar;
- a clinical psychologist;
- a senior nurse;
- a community psychiatric nurse;
- a clinical pharmacist;
- an occupational therapist;
- a social worker; and
- a secretary.

In addition, the teams may include students or other practitioners on undergraduate or postgraduate health and social care training courses.

Forensic case managers, who work within the NHS Specialised Services Agency, may also attend clinical team meetings to review and discuss plans for a patient's potential move on to alternative placements.

Core group meetings

Core group meetings take place in order to facilitate patient care and manage more complex situations that arise, and cannot be fully discussed in the time available within a routine timetabled clinical team meeting. These might involve selected members of the patient's clinical team, and other forensic-service-based workers, who are working with the patient at that time. The meetings provide extra time, to consider in more detail, a patient's treatment strategy and its subsequent implementation by the ward- or unit-based care team.

Information technology

With the appropriate information technology support systems, clinical and other relevant records related to patient care may be held on a computer system. With clinical notes made using a word processor, copies of clinical entries can then be printed at regular intervals and placed in the patient's own hard-copy clinical file. This file is a central record and contains all the notes made by the various disciplines as a record of their work. This then is a *multidisciplinary* document, which can be stored in the nursing office on a hospital residential unit or in a medical records department.

In addition to the maintenance of clinical notes, this form of system also allows for the generation and management of CPA documentation. There may, therefore, be a template for this document, which all disciplines are expected to contribute to at various points, during the patient's care pathway.

Interagency working collaboration

Clinical teams will develop their own links with local health and social care agencies, which create the framework for interagency working. The interface between the clinical team and their respective catchment area services provides an opportunity to discuss matters of clinical practice and service development. It also provides an opportunity to personalise a service when teams meet to present and consider joint working arrangements. Each discipline can meet with counterparts from their own professional group and others, and build up more detailed joint working arrangements, which reflect local requirements.

Multidisciplinary duty 'out-of-hours' system

Whether a forensic service provides so-called parallel or integrated care for outpatients, there may be a 24-hour system of duty cover provided throughout the year by medical, nursing and social work staff, based at the secure unit. This facility may provide solely for patients who are receiving direct follow-up from the forensic service, but may also involve advice on other clinical or related matters to other hospitals.

In the case of patients being followed up by the forensic team, this arrangement may largely depend on and take account of the care plan, which will indicate the patient's needs and, at times, of course, may be what action is to be taken, for instance, in the event of a suspected relapse. The out-of-hours service is staffed by practitioners on a rota, who may not be members of the same clinical team that is responsible for the patients care on a day-to-day basis, illustrating the obvious value of an accessible, comprehensive system of recording and retrieving information.

MULTIDISCIPLINARY WORKING THROUGH THE CARE PROGRAMME APPROACH

One model of practice

This is dealt with in two parts. Part one considers the way the team might organise itself to manage its caseload, from the point of referral of a patient through to follow-up, after leaving the service, reflecting the policy of continuity of care. The second part describes the processes of working with a particular patient whose case represents some of the main issues that a team may deal with as part of the delivery of a forensic mental health care service, and how this relates to the CPA.

Background

The multidisciplinary clinical team meets weekly and is usually chaired by the consultant forensic psychiatrist. The chair follows an agenda, which is circulated in advance by the team's secretary. The agenda itself follows an agreed format. The format is dealt with in some detail because it illustrates how the team works within the framework of the CPA.

Referrals

This area of team activity reflects the process of *interagency* working and the relationships, which have been built up between the clinical team and community, or other hospital-based services. Other mental health service clinicians and workers are usually the referring agents, although this varies.

Patients are normally referred to the team's consultant by:

- consultants/specialist registrars from other health care settings;
- prison health care staff;
- general practitioners;
- patients' solicitors (criminal proceedings).

In addition, the team's clinical psychologist receives referrals from solicitors, for example, seeking a psychological assessment on their client or from National Probation Service colleagues as part of specific liaison work. These referrals are listed as part of the team's activities, although the actual clinical activity may only require the intervention of the team's psychologist. The inclusion is meant to make each team member aware of a patient's contact with the team in case there is further wider involvement and, in addition, it provides an opportunity to discuss issues informally that the patient's situation is presenting and if there is a need for intervention from one of the other team members.

All referred cases appear on the team's agenda in order to consider the reasons for referral, and action to be taken, and by whom, in order to monitor the patient's progress until the agreed intervention has been completed. This could include selected members of the clinical team meeting the referrer to discuss 'on site' the patient's situation in more detail and offer advice on what may be provided to manage the challenges being presented. This activity is offered as an empowering experience to help colleagues understand that their service may be capable of providing the care required, if different strategies are adopted, thus avoiding possible admission to the forensic service. It is about the sharing of professional experiences and expertise, and underlines the importance of interagency collaboration between health and social care systems to maintain people in the most appropriate service. This is one of the principles set out in the Reed Review (Department of Health and Home Office, 1992) referred to in a Social Services Inspectorate publication (Department of Health, 1995): patients should be cared for 'under conditions of no greater security than is justified by the degree of danger they present to themselves or others . . .'

Outpatient reviews

All the team's outpatients are reviewed on a regular basis. This takes two forms: the first is within one of the weekly clinical team meetings when time is set aside to review all outpatients and their progress and any specific matters arising. Patients do not attend this particular review. The review is based on reports, verbal and written, presented by team members who are actively involved in implementing the activities set out in the patient's care plan.

The second form of review is the outpatient CPA case conference, that is, an individual case conference, to which the patient, carers and others are invited, and which takes place to review and, if necessary, revise the care plan.

Inpatients

Patients who are acutely mentally ill are reviewed at least once a week. These people are normally receiving treatment on one of the admission/assessment units. Patients who have settled and are not showing signs of active mental illness are reviewed fortnightly. These people are typically accommodated on one of the rehabilitation residential units.

All 'inpatient' patients are presented by a member of nursing staff who should, ideally, be their patient's key worker. Nursing reports are expected to mention the patient's mental state, behaviour, progress and significant events since last review, and patient requests, plus nursing staff recommendations. This report, which is usually the first to be presented at the team meeting, is then followed by other team member's reports, either verbal or written. Each member of the team is invited to comment on the work they are undertaking, and express views about other aspects of the patient's care and treatment. This is part of the team's joint responsibility and accountability for its clinical management of patients.

All inpatients have a case conference held on them in accordance with the CPA and based on agreed practice. The first formal review, an admission case conference, would usually be held within the first 6 weeks of admission. This should include, where possible, the patient's family, and other health and social services workers who may have previous knowledge of the individual's mental health problems. The team's social worker will prepare reports, which set out the social circumstances. The other disciplines will carry out similar activities in an effort to produce written reports, which make up a comprehensive document that is amended, if necessary, in subsequent meetings. Patients and their families, and carers are encouraged to submit their own reports with assistance from the nursing staff and/or the social worker. The team have created their own form, which invites patients and carers to write about what they think is important for the team to consider in relation to the patient's mental state, psychiatric history or other possible explanations for the person's apparent mental health problems. It is acknowledged that a patient's or carer's literacy skills may make this a difficult exercise, which is approached with sensitivity and awareness that, in addition to any other deficits, the first language of the patient or carer may not be English. If necessary, the forms may be completed by a member of staff.

Case example 1

A 28-year-old man was serving a prison sentence when he became mentally unwell. He was transferred to a medium-secure unit towards the end of his prison sentence. He had expected to be released from prison and allowed to go home. He did not accept that he had mental health problems, and was understandably distressed when he realised that he was being transferred from prison to a psychiatric hospital where he would experience a further period of detention.

His transfer from prison to a medium-secure unit troubled the patient and his family. They had many questions to ask about his situation. The admission case conference provided a forum for their questions to be raised, although they were not necessarily answered to the patient and his family's satisfaction. He and some members of his family attended his admission case conference. They were invited to read the reports that had been written by the members of the team and to listen to the nursing key worker's report.

The patient's legal representative attended the case conference to assist him in asking questions about his current care and plans for his future care. His family was likewise invited to contribute to the discussion.

This man was diagnosed as suffering from a mental illness and in need of treatment. He was informed about the reasons why it was felt he needed treatment in conditions of medium security. He did not accept that he suffered from mental health problems. His family accepted that he was not well but could not see the justification in his detention in a secure hospital.

The admission case conference provided an opportunity to openly discuss the professional views of team members and take into account the views of the patient and his family. In this case, he and his family expressed their dissatisfaction with the arrangements. Admission case conferences do not necessarily end with agreement between patient and care team. They do, however, provide opportunities to explain to the patient and their family the reasons for the planned interventions.

Risk assessment

At this stage, that is, the admission case conference, the process of completing a standard risk assessment instrument begins. This process includes two or more team members ideally from different disciplines analysing the data against the questions posed.

The frequency of subsequent case conferences during the inpatient phase is determined by a patient's progress.

Ethnicity cultural and religious matters

Secure psychiatric and forensic services have responsibility for the provision of forensic mental health care services to a wide variety of different catchment areas. The demographic profile of the potential patient group may also vary. There may be diversity of ethnicity, religious and socioeconomic groups within the total population. In some areas of the country, the percentage of black patients is approximately 35%.

Clinical teams, which may, in the main, be composed mainly of white professional workers, must be aware of the over-representation of black patients. The multiprofessional approach allows for this situation to be considered and addressed where possible and practicable. The models of intervention include the *biopsychosocial* assessment process. This model provides for a holistic assessment of a patient's individual set of circumstances. It assumes direct engagement between team members, and the patient and family to assess and understand what the particular circumstances are. This process provides opportunities to identify personal matters that are important to the patient in terms of his culture, religion or faith, in addition to his health and social care needs. Information gathered in this process is fed back into clinical team meetings and case conferences to amend, if necessary, the patient's care plan. This approach attempts to deal with, and positively overcome, any discriminatory practices during the period of inpatient care and follow-up in the community.

Efforts should always be made to engage with the patient's own community-based links to consider what cultural and religious matters need to be addressed whilst the patient is disconnected from previous support systems. The team must recognise the importance of cultural awareness in terms of whether the presentation of a patient's 'mental health problems' is consistent with belief systems held within a particular religion or culture. This is a problematic area dealt with by Fernando (1991, 1995) and Rack (1982), who write about the experiences of black patients and south Asian patients in English psychiatric systems.

The multidisciplinary team should also appreciate the individuality of its patients, and the right they have to be treated with respect and in a dignified manner. This should be enshrined in service policies that reflect the need and directive to think more positively about cultural diversity.

Victim perspective

The work of a multidisciplinary team must also take into account the perspective of the victim. This is an obvious point, in terms of information gathering to assess risk, but this is not the only team activity that relates to that aspect.

Multidisciplinary working in a forensic service has to balance the rights and needs of a patient with the rights/needs of the victim, potential or real. This situation can, and frequently does, create conflicts that have to be resolved if the patient is to be allowed to live in the community successfully once more. The resolution of these conflicts may not, however, be in the gift of the clinical team.

Case example 2

The patient was a white male who suffered from longstanding mental health problems. He had been living with his parents who had cared for him during his numerous episodes of acute illness. He developed a belief that there was a conspiracy to harm him. He became completely consumed by this and he felt compelled to act. He attacked his mother in the expectation that he would be taken to court where he could explain to the authorities his belief about the conspiracy against him.

His mother was seriously injured and required hospitalisation. The patient was found to be suffering from another acute psychotic episode. He was admitted to a medium-secure unit for assessment and treatment.

The man's mother understood her son's mental health problems and knew that he was acting on the basis of his abnormal beliefs when he attacked her. Her views, as his mother and as a victim, were taken fully into account when the care plan was initially constructed and revised in the light of his progress.

The clinical team began working with the patient more at his pace of recovery and the pace of his mother, as she came to terms with what had happened to her, and made efforts to reconstruct her life. She had been severely traumatised, emotionally and physically, by the incident.

The patient's mother's views had to be taken into account. She loved her son but feared for her own personal safety. The team had a double challenge. Firstly, to respond to the challenge of treating his condition, thus substantially reducing his risk of reoffending, and secondly, to work with his mother to make her feel safe and help her understand that the treatment he was receiving would reduce his risk of harming her and others. The team had to organise itself to make these activities run in parallel to ensure that the patient and his mother felt in control of their respective situations.

The patient eventually made a substantial recovery and his mother's confidence grew to a point where she felt comfortable when he made home visits to see her.

A multidisciplinary team must, of course, be aware that its work with a patient will be open at various stages to the scrutiny of others, as the patient passes through the legal process and mental health system. These include the Home Office Mental Health Unit, the Mental Health Review Tribunal, Mental Health Act Commission and other outside agencies.

There are points in the patient's care pathway, where the work of treatment and rehabilitation may bring the patient into contact with the victim or the victim's family. It has to be stressed that a multidisciplinary clinical team does not routinely deal with victim work in situations of 'stranger attack'. However, in many cases, the victim is in some way related to the patient, typically a partner or close member of the family. In these situations, contact takes place between various professional forensic personnel and the victim, or the victim's family, as they visit the patient. Specific members of a multidisciplinary team will have their own formal contact with the victim and family to undertake their own assessments, which include whether there is a need for support from the forensic mental health care or other services.

In the situation of an attack on a stranger, contacts may be made with National Probation Victim Support Units for guidance on victim perspectives and views about rehabilitation plans in terms of community visits and placements.

Media attention

The team must also take into account the possibility of adverse media attention affecting treatment and patient rehabilitation. As previously stated, this creates difficulties for implementing care plans, particularly in 'high-profile' cases, which have, for instance, attracted national media coverage. It is a 'fact of life' that practitioners have learnt to accept and one that patients in these circumstances have to come to terms with.

Home Office (Mental Health Unit)

In England and Wales, the Home Office occupies a key position in terms of progressing a patient's programme of treatment and rehabilitation. This position relates to patients who are compulsorily detained as remanded or transferred prisoners, and those subject to hospital orders with restrictions on discharge.

The Home Office's Mental Health Unit makes its decisions based on the information provided by the clinical team and ministerial directions. This serves to underline the extent to which mental health care services in certain situations are politicised and subject to political dogma. This is another example of how forensic multidisciplinary team working in the CPA differs from that of general psychiatric services in terms of professional autonomy, that is, freedom to practise without reference to or permission from non-clinical authorities.

Interagency working

This is established with local health and social care agencies as soon as the patient is admitted. Efforts are made to have contacts with local services to begin the working relationship of partnership to include joint assessment and co-working. This is not always easy to achieve within a regionally organised service because of the distances to the patient's local areas in some cases. However, every effort should be made to gather local service information, which may be of use to the team.

Pre-discharge planning

At this stage, there should be an informed understanding of the social and health care needs of the patient and, where appropriate, carers. Previous case conferences and ongoing weekly team discussions should have identified what services are required to enable the patient to move on from the medium secure unit. This planned progression may be into the community at large, but may also involve transfer to other specialist inpatient health care services.

As part of the interagency arrangements, local health and social care services should be working with the multidisciplinary team to either directly provide from their own resources, or commission from others the services required to support the community care plan. This aspect of care planning is crucial because it involves increasing amounts of exposure of the patient into the community and can be a stressful period for all those concerned.

At the pre-discharge stage, the multidisciplinary team must ensure that all interested parties and stakeholders are aware of the care plan and that they support it. This position is reinforced, through the process of a pre-discharge meeting, which should include all those people who are identified within the care plan.

The care plan as part of the overall CPA document is presented in draft form, for discussion and possible amendment. It will include a summary of the risk assessment, based on the data gathered since the patient's admission, dealing with, in some detail, history of offending behaviours, and any history of violence. Team members will state their intended interventions in support of the care plan. Early warning signs of deterioration are noted along with what action is to be taken in the event of relapse. The care plan will also have a section that allows a patient, carer or provider to express their views, noting any disagreement with the plan and 'measures of success' to monitor the outcomes of the plan. A copy is made available for the patient, carer and provider for their information, which is signed by them.

Case example 3

This case demonstrates how team members approached the processes of assessment, treatment and rehabilitation for the patient, and how this collaborative exercise, which included interagency working, enabled him to return to live in the community successfully.

The patient was a single white male. He had a history of mental health problems, and had been treated and supported by his local health and social care services. He was diagnosed as suffering from depression associated with post-traumatic stress disorder (PTSD) and personality problems. He also had a history of ideas of self-harm and had attempted suicide on several occasions by taking analgesics. Following each of these attempts he was admitted for inpatient treatment but discharged within a few days. He had a chequered career in terms of employment. His mental health problems prevented him from working full time. He attended a local sheltered workshop. At the time of his index offence, he was living with his parents who were concerned about his mental health. They offered their support to help him cope with his difficulties and tried to deal with any crises he presented. They were dissatisfied with the lack of support from local services.

The patient was referred to the forensic services following an incident in which he took a knife from his parent's house and threatened a neighbour. After this incident, he walked into a local library where he was subsequently arrested by armed police officers. He was taken into police custody and examined by a forensic medical examiner, was charged and appeared in court, where he was remanded in custody. In prison, he appeared depressed and suicidal. He was assessed and transferred to a medium-secure unit under the provisions of Sections 48/49 of the Mental Health Act 1983.

In the medium-secure unit he recovered from his low mood but experienced 'flashbacks' associated with his PTSD. In the course of assessment, he was diagnosed as suffering from personality problems.

When this man appeared in court again, he pleaded guilty to the offences. He was given a Probation Order with conditions of medical treatment. Following a further period as an inpatient, he was discharged to live in a supervised hostel for people recovering from mental illness. After a period of follow-up by his clinical team, his care was transferred back to local services.

This case summary will now be considered in terms of multidisciplinary team working and the CPA. Following his arrest, it was noted during the initial police investigations that the patient had a history of mental health problems, and had presented with bouts of severe depression and suicidal thinking. He could have been diverted away from custody at the point when he was in police custody or after his court appearance. His local health and social care services, however, were unable to provide him with an inpatient bed. In view of the nature of his offence and the perceived risk of self-harm, it was decided to detain him in custody and remand him to prison to be kept under close supervision.

He was subsequently referred to the forensic clinical team. Arrangements were made for an urgent medical and nursing assessment, which took place in prison. Following this, he was admitted to the medium-secure unit and was placed in the intensive care unit on special continuous observations. His condition required urgent medical and nursing interventions to start the process of treating his depression and preventing him from committing suicide.

The patient's local health and social care services were contacted by the clinical team's psychiatrist and social worker within a provisionally agreed protocol concerning notification of admissions and request for information. These arrangements formed part of the interagency agreements to monitor patient's placements and progress.

Local services notified the clinical team that they had received a complaint from his parents about their son's treatment. This appeared to restrict the amount of information that was available, and the comments that local services workers could make about the patient's condition and how it had been managed. The clinical team's social worker and community psychiatric nurse visited his parents. The visit served many purposes. The initial contact was an opportunity for families to vent their feelings, and share their concerns and worries about what had actually happened. The social worker and community psychiatric nurse allowed them to express their feelings and to try to come to terms with what had happened. In the course of the interview, information was also gathered about the patient's personal and developmental history, and family attitudes towards what had taken place. This was an important part of the risk assessment process in terms of predicting how the family would behave and whether they could be relied upon to work with the clinical team when the patient was again living in the community.

It became apparent in the early stages of this man's admission that he had suffered long-term mental health problems, which included depression, PTSD and personality-related difficulties. Within the CPA, the clinical team drew up a care plan, which focused in each of these specific areas. The consultant forensic psychiatrist prescribed antidepressant medication after a discussion with medical colleagues about the patient's mental state and what would be appropriate. The team's psychologist agreed to coordinate work with the effects of the PTSD. This included individual sessions with the family. The patient wanted to share with his parents the events that led up to the trauma he had experienced. He previously felt unable to talk to them about it. The psychologist worked with him to examine what the difficulties were and how he could deal with these. The social worker talked to the parents about his difficulties in talking to them about past trauma, which had made him depressed. This work led to family meetings, which included the patient, his parents, the key worker, the team's social worker and the psychologist. Over several meetings, he was eventually able to disclose what had taken place and how bad he felt about what had happened to him. This intervention was helped by the medication lifting his mood and he was able to focus on the matters that had concerned him. He felt more able to engage and consequently became less withdrawn.

In the implementation of this care plan, the multidisciplinary team was able to assess his mental state and to begin to develop a formulation concerning his risk and how it might be managed. The team continued to gather information.

The patient was charged with offences relating to possession of an offensive weapon and threats to kill. He potentially faced a prison sentence. Both he and his parents understood the severity of the charges and the possible outcome, but agreed that he was unwell at the time and did not intend any harm to anybody. He had, he said, threatened to harm others in the hope that the police would kill him. The neighbour had written a statement, which indicated that she believed that he was going to carry out his threat to harm her. People in the library had similar concerns about their personal safety.

On the one hand, there was clear evidence that the patient was unwell at the time of the offence and was not fully in control of his actions. He was depressed and wanted to die by being killed by the police. On the other hand, the multidisciplinary team had to take into account the views of the victim, and the public's perception, as reported by the media. In this situation, the neighbour was a stranger and, therefore, not immediately accessible to the clinical team workers, who were required to work with the local victim support unit. The care plan could not be exclusively patient focused because the rehabilitation plan, as it related to the patient's exposure to the community, could have had adverse effects on the victim and patient.

The patient had to wait several months before his eventual court appearance. During this time, he made a significant recovery in his mental health in terms of his depression. The joint work with him and his family had led to improvement in his PTSD. There remained personality difficulties, which had been identified by the psychologist who formed the view that he had developed an inner strength and coping strategies to manage these. Through multidisciplinary team discussions, it was concluded that the patient was no longer detainable under the Mental Health Act and that, when he appeared in court, the team could not recommend a hospital order. In anticipation of this, the patient was referred to the National Probation Service for assessment of his suitability for a probation order with conditions of medical treatment.

The team had been pursuing a care plan within the CPA, which attempted to assess the patient's health and social care needs in a comprehensive and systematic way, and in one that could be understood by him and his parents. In the course of working with him and his parents, the team had been able to develop a clearer picture of this man's mental health problems and how they should be managed. This understanding was the result of weekly meetings to discuss his progress, and to receive reports from team members about their work as well as case conferences, which included his parents, his legal representative, and local health and social care workers. The next phase of work was to plan for his return to the community.

The patient was transferred to a rehabilitation unit within the service and his risk of self-harm had significantly reduced after his court appearance, when his case had been dealt with. He felt relieved that he would not have to serve a prison sentence and that the work on his mental health problems could carry on with the same multidisciplinary team. He was more able to participate in a wider range of occupational therapy activities.

As previously stated, the care plan and the CPA had to move forward with caution because of the position with regard to the victim. The Probation Service inquiries through the victim support unit made it quite clear that the patient could not return to his parent's home address. The alternative was a residential placement because the team was of the opinion that he still required support to help him settle back down into the community. A care manager was identified and he undertook the research into available and suitable accommodation.

The patient was eventually found a placement in a supported hostel for people with mental health problems. This was offered after the accommodation providers had carried out their own assessment and had read, with the patient's consent, the team's clinical notes, care plan, case conference reports, etc.

The patient was later referred to the local services covering his new home address. There was understandable concern. Further reports, letters of clarification and joint meetings took place before he was accepted for transfer. In consultation with hostel staff, the process was overseen by the forensic services, which worked in partnership with the original local services as they progressed through the process of transfer to his new local services. Local police were also involved in the planning because of his offending behaviours. A multiagency public protection panel meeting was held to examine any potential risks posed.

The patient's original local services and the key representatives from the forensic team withdrew, leaving the National Probation Service and local health and social care services to provide the agreed package of aftercare/CPA services.

Summary

This case provides an example of forensic multidisciplinary team working within the clear framework of CPA. The team had in place systems, which comprehensively assessed health and social care needs in consultation and partnership with carers and local services. This took place against a background of developing interagency arrangements, which facilitated the coordinated delivery of services, open communication and cooperation. It took into account the victim perspective and any public protection issues. The risk assessment and management formulation concluded that it was appropriate for the patient to move on to live in the community.

References

Bailey D (2000) Care planning and care coordination in mental health. In: At the core of mental health: key issues for practitioners, managers and mental health trainers, Chapter 8. London: Pavilion

CPA Association (2001) The CPA handbook. Chesterfield: The CPA Association Walton Hospital

Department of Health (1990) HC 90 23/ LASL (90) The Care Programme Approach for people with mental illness referred to the specialist psychiatric services. London: HMSO

Department of Health (1995a) The Health of the Nation Building Bridges: a guide to arrangements for the care of severe mentally ill people. London: HMSO

Department of Health (1995b) Social Services Inspectorate mentally disordered offenders: improving services. London: HMSO

Department of Health (1996) An audit pack for monitoring the Care Programme Approach: background and explanatory notes. NHS Executive. London: HMSO

Department of Health (1999a) Mental health national service framework: modern standards and service models. London: HMSO

Department of Health (2003) Developing services for carers and families of people with mental illness. London: HMSO

Department of Health and Home Office (1992) Review of health and social services for mentally disordered offenders and others requiring similar services. London: HMSO

Department of Health and Social Services Inspectorate (1995) Social services department and the CPA: an inspection report. London: HMSO

Fernando S (1991) Mental health race and culture. London: Macmillan Press

Fernando S (1995) Mental health in multi ethnic society: a multidisciplinary handbook. London: Routledge

Ministry of Health (1962) The hospital plan for England and Wales, cmnd 1604. London: HMSO

Rack P (1982) Race, culture and mental disorder. London: Routledge

Reith M (1998) Community care tragedies: a practice guide to the mental health inquiries. Birmingham: Venture Press

Sheppard D (1996) Learning the lessons, 2nd edn. London: Zito Trust

Social Services Inspectorate and NHS Executive (1999) Effective care co-ordination in the metal health services: modernising the Care Programme Approach (a policy booklet). London: HMSO

Chapter **8**

Risk assessment: a multidisciplinary approach to estimating harmful behaviour in mentally disordered offenders

Jason Jones and Chris Plowman

CHAPTER CONTENTS

INTRODUCTION

The assessment of risk, particularly of harmful behaviour towards others, is now a vital and mandatory element of effective multidisciplinary working in mental health services. It is no longer sufficient to assess and treat mental illness and other forms of mental disorder, and increasingly, mental health services have become driven by an agenda of public protection. Within the UK, there continues to be change, with the advent of services for individuals with dangerous and severe personality disorder, and the emphasis on risk will extend. As such, clinicians are being required to become experts in the area of risk assessment. Sadly, there are inherent problems with this for the mental health practitioner. There are few measures of risk that are easily accessible without extensive knowledge of the background literature. Information that is routinely gathered during clinical assessment and other interventions does not always lend itself naturally to illuminate areas of risk. The completion of risk assessments is reassuringly time-consuming but equally is a burdensome task for the already encumbered clinician. The process of risk assessment is ongoing, frequently requiring discussion, updating and specific action. Furthermore, the costs for clinicians, of making accurate or inaccurate assessments of risk, are high and not easily shared with others.

The aim of this chapter is to address some of these concerns. By beginning with a review of available assessments of risk of violence, the means of gathering information within a multidisciplinary context will then be considered. The chapter concludes with some guidance on managing the onus and process of risk assessment.

THE STATE OF THE ART

Risk prediction remains more art than science. However, the last 10 years has seen an increasing trend towards developing more valid and reliable means of assessing risk. Before the advent of such methods, it was typical for clinician judgement to be the main method of risk assessment of violence. Such judgements were often, but not necessarily, based on an in-depth knowledge of the individual concerned. However, such judgements were also vulnerable to the influence of biased assumptions, potentially inherent and diverse across different disciplines. Consider for a moment the relative importance attributed to mental state by psychiatrists and psychologists. Individuals might both agree about the importance of understanding mental state in risk assessment, but the attributed weight given to this factor by members of each profession is likely to vary substantially. It is because of factors such as this that clinical judgement-based risk assessments came under considerable scrutiny. Early studies (Steadman et al., 1993) found that clinicians often predicted risk with little accuracy. Unsurprisingly, clinicians erred towards overprediction (Lidz et al., 1993).

Mainly owing to the political imperatives for clinicians to develop risk assessment strategies, the research in this area has taken a predominantly scientific approach. This has led to a focus on actuarial measures of risk of violence in people diagnosed with mental illness. However, there remains an emphasis on clinical judgement. Hence, the present plethora of risk assessment guides and strategies mean that there is a blending of scientific rigour with the artistry of clinical judgement. One invariably impacts on the other and so, for the time being, risk assessment relies on science but remains more of an art. This is important to remember, in that science, supported by impressive statistics, can mislead the busy clinicians into thinking that a prediction has been made. However, with the tools currently available, risk can only ever be estimated. Thus, a person's actual risk of violence can never be known. With this caveat in mind, the remainder of this section will consider what science has to offer.

RECENT TRENDS IN RISK ASSESSMENT

Over the last 20 years, the major developments in risk assessment have occurred from within North American clinical and research facilities. Careful documentation combined with the application of novel statistical procedures have led to the development of a series of actuarial measures of risk of violence. These and other contributions are considered next.

Actuarial measures of risk of violence

The process of risk assessment is undoubtedly enriched by the availability of actuarial data. Frequently, within routine clinical practice, a patient may cause anxieties amongst a clinical team, raising their estimates of the potential for harmful behaviour. Actuarial data and knowledge of the relevant base rates of harmful behaviour provide an anchor against the force of this bias. Actuarial measures and their data refer to instruments or statistics based on what is actually known about violent or harmful behaviour. In other words, from previous case examples, we can examine the distribution, characteristics, influencing variables and outcomes of previous harmful behaviour.

An exhaustive explication of the range of actuarial measures of risk of violence is beyond the scope of this chapter. Some excellent resources exist nevertheless, and the interested reader is directed to those for a fuller consideration of the development and application of actuarial measures of risk of violence in people with mental disorders (e.g. Webster et al., 1997; Quinsey et al., 1998; Monahan et al., 2001).

The HCR-20 (Webster et al., 1997) is a Canadian-based guide to violence risk assessment. The title stands for the three sections that make up the assessment: history, current clinical presentation, and future risk judgements. The history section makes up half of the 20 items on the HCR-20, and draws heavily on the known literature of actuarial predictors of violent behaviour. The items are selected by the expert authors, rather than derived from purely empirical means. Initial use of the HCR-20 has been very popular, allowing some degree of freedom from numerical estimates and providing a comprehensive source of risky behaviours. The HCR-20 is completed by a review of the files, usually considered within the context of multidisciplinary discussion.

No one profession is better than any other, yet each will have strengths for specific items. For instance, a psychiatrist, community psychiatric nurse or inpatient ward nurse might best be placed to comment on an individual's active symptoms, diagnosis or current mental state. Similarly, a social worker can offer a valued opinion on the social context available for future discharge, such as exposure to destabilisers, and whether realistic plans have been made and agreed with the individual. A psychologist is usually best placed to comment on the assessment of psychopathy, or offer comment on early maladjustment or childhood difficulties. As such, the HCR-20 is a good example of a multidisciplinary risk assessment.

There are some important considerations to be made when deciding on the use of the HCR-20. The first is the use of scores. In the initial version of the HCR-20, a three-point scoring system is applied, with higher scores reflecting higher risk. This has the disadvantage of reducing the effort taken to complete an HCR-20 to a single number, against which few if any norms are available. Thus, if a multidisciplinary team completes an HCR-20 on a patient and a score of 30 is yielded, it is difficult to ascertain to what extent this should be considered to reflect risk. Therefore, it is best advised to use the numeric system merely as a guide within routine clinical practice. A new version of the HCR-20 is available where the coding has been replaced by a simpler system of clarifying whether the item is present or absent.

A full HCR-20 is typically a time-consuming exercise, which from conceptualisation to completion can take a minimum of 6 hours. In order to ensure reward from such effort, it is important to summarise or formulate an individual's risk adequately. Here attention can be paid to the nature of the violence, the context, the cost and the victim characteristics of potential future violence. Guidance is not available for this within the standard HCR-20 documentation; however, this can be supplemented by other available guides (e.g. Moore, 1996). This requires additional work but often proves to be one of the most valuable components of multidisciplinary discussion.

The HCR-20 is fundamentally a framework that guides the collection of information pertinent to an assessment of risk of violence. As such, it relies on the quality of the information available about the individual. Hence, despite the presence of actuarial factors, it remains susceptible to some of the same biases and limitations of risk assessments based on pure clinical judgement.

The violence risk appraisal guide (VRAG; Quinsey et al., 1998) and its accompanying sex offender risk appraisal guide (SORAG) are purer actuarial measures than the HCR-20. Each comprises a series of items, derived from an empirical analysis of mentally disordered offenders who have been assessed and treated at Pentanguishene State Hospital in Canada. Therefore, the items comprising the VRAG are based on the characteristics of individuals detained in maximum secure care. Owing to the statistical derivation of the VRAG, the items are weighted for their respective relevance to the prediction of risk. Once completed, an overall risk score is yielded that can be checked against the normative data available for that original population. Two estimates are available, one for the likelihood of violence occurring within the next 7 years of opportunity (i.e. postdischarge or release) and one for within the next 10 years of opportunity. Thus, a probability is ascertained that is meant to reflect the risk of violence occurring.

Whilst there is something reassuring about being given a probability statistic of violence occurring, it is often very difficult to ascertain how this actually can affect clinical practice and subsequent risk management. Supposing for a moment that VRAGs are completed on two patients appealing for discharge from a secure hospital. One patient's score indicates that there is a 72% chance of violence recurring within the next 7 years and the other patient's score indicates that there is a 56% chance of violence recurring within the next 10 years. Although, in the first example, the percentage is higher, to what extent is this likely to impact on the risk management of the individual? It is yet to be determined whether a multidisciplinary team would be better advised by one statistic than the other. The timescales provided offer little help. It is unusual for individuals to be intensively managed for periods of 7–10 years, particularly if they are mentally well during that time. Hence the service demand implications need to be carefully considered, as it could quite easily be a situation where forensic follow-up is indicated for up to 7 years. This provides scant hope for already overburdened services and even less hope for the individual about whom the judgement has been made.

A further consideration with the VRAG is the data upon which it is based. Pentanguishene is a Canadian maximum-secure facility for individuals with diagnoses of severe mental health problems and/or personality disorders. It adopted a treatment strategy markedly different to that employed generally within forensic mental health services in the UK. Thus, it is important to consider how relevant comparisons to the population studied actually are.

The level of service inventory (LSI-R; Andrews and Bonta, 1995) was developed to operationalise the balance between the identification of risk markers and the related further needs for service input. Hereby, the LSI-R marks the first structured attempt to establish the relationship between risk and needs assessment. The risk markers are broadly similar to those in other measures, with emphasis particularly given to previous criminality. However, the LSI-R addresses a broad range of offending behaviour and, therefore, does not only offer an estimate of risk for violence. Some novel additions were included in this measure that are worthy of comment. A detailed consideration is required of the nature of an individual's interactions with peers and authority figures within education and employment. Importance is also attributed to the assessment of the individual's financial situation and accommodation. Furthermore, pointed questions are asked of the nature of an individual's peer relationships generally within the community. For example, if an individual has a number of criminal acquaintances or friends, this is considered important and might indicate an area for future work.

The LSI-R has been used in a series of normative studies (e.g. Andrews, 1982; Bonta and Motiuk, 1985; Andrews et al., 1986). Consequently, data are available for male and female inmates, in addition to individuals being managed on probation orders within the community. As such, it retains good flexibility and applicability. However, it is likely that this measure is restricted when applied to mentally disordered offenders. At present, no normative data are available, and medical diagnosis is not considered a key risk marker on the LSI-R. This appears to again contradict the data used on the creation of the HCR-20 and the VRAG. However, in individuals where mental health diagnosis is less associated with risk, this provides a useful adjunct to the risk assessment process.

PSYCHOPATHY AND RISK OF VIOLENCE

The concept of psychopathy has long been associated with risk of violence (Hemphill et al., 1998). Psychopathy is usually classified as a disorder of personality. Standard definitions include problems with emotional, behavioural and interpersonal factors. Emotionally, psychopaths are considered to be lacking in empathy and remorse, and are cunning, manipulative and grandiose. At the behavioural level, psychopaths are thought to be impulsive, disregarding of societal conventions and prone to high-risk behaviours. Interpersonally, psychopaths are thought to be dominant, unable to form close emotional attachments to others, and are superficial. Not surprisingly, therefore, individuals classified as being psychopathic are those most often associated with a proneness to use violence or commit acts of crime (Hare, 1993). Unfortunately, there is a lack of clarity and distinction when considering the differences between psychopathy and antisocial personality disorder (ASPD) (Thomas-Peter and Jones, 2004).

The assessment of psychopathy is best aided by the use of the Hare psychopathy checklist (revised, PCL-R; or screening version, PCL-SV). Primarily developed and tested in Canada and North America (Hare, 1991), the PCL-R is an established predictor of risk for violence and general criminal recidivism. Hemphill et al. (1998) found that PCL-R scores alone were strongly associated with future violent behaviour and a better predictor of violent recidivism than actuarial data alone. In a civil psychiatric population, Steadman et al. (1998) have shown that the PCL-SV is the single best predictor of postdischarge violence compared with 133 potential other predictors. Similarly, in a UK sample, the PCL-SV was found to be a good predictor of violence within institutions (Doyle et al., 2002). UK predictive validity was also established for the PCL-R amongst mentally disordered offenders (Gray et al., 2003). Therefore, the inclusion of the PCL-R or the PCL-SV within-risk assessments remains important and may augment the assessment of risk.

EFFECTIVENESS OF CURRENT METHODS

The original conclusions reached by Monahan and Steadman (1994) still remain important. They noted that the field of risk assessments was prone to four major methodological limitations, namely, weak criterion variables for violence, constricted validation samples, inadequacy of predictors and unsynchronised research efforts. Unfortunately, none of the formal risk assessment measures considered earlier adequately address these major methodological considerations. Although all have established good criterion variables for violence with satisfactory prediction adequacy, the research efforts have remained unsynchronised. Consequently, only limited data are available about the validity of these measures across diverse populations. Therefore, it is essential for the clinician, when conducting a risk assessment, to go beyond the standard measures. The remainder of this chapter hopes to enable that process further. First, ranges of factors are discussed that are commonly overlooked in risk assessments but which may retain some clinical utility. Second, the art of risk assessment within multidisciplinary working is considered.

VIOLENCE IN MENTALLY DISORDERED OFFENDERS

It is important to note that not all mentally disordered offenders are prone to violent or dangerous behaviour, just as not all dangerous offenders are mentally disordered. As far back as 1975, Tennent suggested that three types of relationship may exist between violence and mental disorder. Firstly, that violence can occur as a result of the mental disorder, in which case treatment of the disorder would be expected to ameliorate the dangerous behaviour. Secondly, that violence may occur in the mentally disordered but that treatment of the mental disorder may not reduce the behaviour. Lastly, that violence may occur in the absence of mental disorder. Somewhat wryly, Tennent notes that these categories, especially the first two, tend to merge in legal terms. Thus, society appears to be moving further towards the 'criminalisation of the mentally ill' (see Rice and Harris, 1997, for a detailed review). Thus, this appears to fly in the face of the revised findings of Steadman et al. (1998) who, in contradiction to the seminal research of Swanson et al. (1990) found that 'psychosis alone' patients were not more dangerous than non-patients. However, they did confirm the earlier research that substance misuse, in the absence of mental disorder, is itself related to violence, but that this effect size increases significantly if substance misuse is combined with psychosis. In the earlier study, they found that the 'psychosis alone' group were three times more likely to be violent within a year, when compared to non-patients. It should be noted, however, that the absolute risk in this group was relatively low (7%) and that those with a diagnosis of alcoholism were 12 times more violent, whilst those with a diagnosis of drug misuse were 16 times more likely to be violent than non-patients. These findings, amongst other actuarial risk reviews, conclude that mental state, in and of itself, is a weaker predictive variable than young age, low social class, unemployment, male gender and previous use of violence. Thus, it is perhaps too soon to say, as stated by Monahan in 1992, that individuals experiencing a mental disorder are at no greater risk of committing a violent act than the general public. This is because, when factors such as social class or substance use are controlled for, it is found that they, in themselves, may be a consequence or even a cause of the mental disorder itself.

PREVALENCE AND IMMINENCE

In light of the constraints addressed earlier, considerable care must be taken in generalising research findings to the clinical field. The results of the MacArthur Risk Assessment Study, the largest best-designed study of violence amongst the mentally disordered to date, was published by Steadman et al. (1998). This examined 1136 male and female patients with mental disorders who were followed up every 10 weeks during their fist year postdischarge from a psychiatric unit. These results were analysed for violence using a comparison group of 519 randomly sampled non-patients from the same census area. Briefly, their main conclusions indicated that substance misuse appeared to be the key variable in determining the prevalence of violence in a mentally disordered population:

- The presence of substance abuse increased both the frequency and severity of the aggressive acts.
- The patient group without substance misuse did not differ from the community control group, without substance use, in the frequency of aggression.
- Patients had symptoms of substance misuse more frequently than community controls.

PREDICTIVE FACTORS

A recent systematic review of risk factors for 'imminent' violence in mental health services concluded that there is no clear consensus on items that would be useful for short-term prediction (Royal College of

Psychiatrists, 1998). However, a range of risk markers exist that are often not included in the standardised risk assessment tools. They are considered here, because, although in broad samples they may have reduced statistical value, it is possible that these issues will need to be considered on an individual basis.

INDIVIDUAL CHARACTERISTICS

Some individual characteristics have consistently been found to relate to violent behaviour. Many of these are common sense and those things that a lay person would consider if asked to make predictions about potentially violent individuals. These would include gender, age, and previous criminal or violent behaviours. Thus, 90% of violence is perpetrated by men (Monahan, 1993), primarily in their late teens or twenties, and whom had been previously convicted of a violent offence. In fact, the latter has been found in the majority of studies to be the most stable of all the predictor variables. However, the presence or absence of previous violence is insufficient, in itself, to aid the prediction. Factors such as the previous offending context, including the environmental, emotional and victim conditions must be taken into account.

Others variables require rather more expertise and sensitivity to assess. Variables such as childhood histories of abuse or neglect are frequently gathered through social services or school reports, whilst the presence or absence of psychopathy, covered in detail previously, requires specialist assessment skills not generally found in community services who have neither the time available nor the training to undertake an assessment of such complexity.

SOCIODEMOGRAPHIC FACTORS

Silver et al. (1999), in following up 293 discharged patients from Pittsburgh, found certain interpersonal variables were associated with violence. They concluded that men were more violent that women, African-Americans were more violent than whites, those with previous arrests for serious crimes, abused alcohol or illicit drugs or who had a diagnosis of ASPD were significantly more violent than those without. However, when economical variables were examined, it was found that those discharged to poor areas were more than twice as likely to be violent as those discharged to wealthier areas. Additionally, certain individual predictors disappeared under the influence of these factors. For example, it was found that African-Americans were no more violent than whites when discharged to richer areas. However, those patients with drug or alcohol problems, or prior arrest or a diagnosed ASPD were significantly more likely to be violent in poorer areas. Similarly, Singleton et al. (1998) found that only 36% of male remand prisoners and 44% of male sentenced prisoners had been employed prior to their incarceration. When considering future placements of patients within the community, it is worthwhile considering the potential effect of placing them in an economically deprived area with little opportunities for employment, as the research evidence suggests this is likely to significantly affect the level of risk the person poses.

CLINICAL AND/OR DIAGNOSTIC FACTORS

These issues would fall under the caveat of risk state rather than risk status. Thus, it is defined as a patient's propensity to act violently at a given time. It is noted to vary according to the person's biological, psychological or social variables. For example, it has been found that individuals with severe psychotic illness are more likely to commit acts of violence when experiencing an acute psychotic episode, including delusions and hallucinations (Link and Stueve, 1994; McNiel, 1994; Modestin and Ammann 1995), or during episodes of substance misuse or non-compliance with medication (Swartz et al., 1998). Additionally, it has been a consistent finding that substance misuse (including alcohol and illicit drugs) is one of the principal predictors of violence in both the mentally disordered and the non-disordered populations. Further, across both populations, the majority of violent crimes are committed by individuals under the influence of alcohol. However, when detailing a risk assessment, it is important to acknowledge the ways in which the alcohol or drug use relates to the violence. For example, the violence may be directly related to the intoxication, but equally may relate to withdrawal effects, acquisitive behaviours or personality changes brought about by long-term use.

SITUATIONAL AND CONTEXTUAL FACTORS

As with clinical and/or diagnostic factors, risk state must be taken into account. Thus, the presence of available weapons or social support may dramatically alter the risk state, and ultimately risk status (Heilbrun, 1997; Kraemer et al., 1997). Howlett (1998) examined the role of treatment non-compliance in homicide inquiries by individuals suffering from a mental illness. He found that nearly two-thirds highlighted medication non-compliance as a major contributory factor in the breakdown of care prior to the homicide. Of further interest are the more recent findings implicating social context and support in the incidence of violence. Thus, Martell et al. (1995), who investigated the association between homelessness, mental disorder and violence, found that the mentally disordered population were 40 times more likely to be homeless when compared to the general population, and were significantly more likely to be arrested and charged for violence.

IMPROVING CLINICIAN-BASED RISK ASSESSMENT

Blumenthal and Lavender (2000) suggest a useful process to adopt when compiling risk assessments. Moore (1996) strongly asserts the necessity to reduce bias and error in clinician-based risk assessments. We have attempted to marry these perspectives with the previous considerations of the actuarial frameworks for risk assessment.

Towards a gold standard

The process of risk assessment should be grounded within a full and detailed history of the individual being assessed. Where possible, this history should cover the range of individual experiences that are considered important by each discipline. The following should be a minimum amount of information on which to begin to base a risk assessment.

1. *Family background.* In particular, note the quality of the relationship with parents (whether biological or other primary caregivers) and siblings. Establish areas of difficulty or conflict during childhood within the family home and surrounding community. Document any experiences of abuse, either as a victim or perpetrator, and where possible, consider the impact of such experiences on the development of the individual.

2. *Educational history.* Describe how the individual adapted to their educational environment. Consider the quality of relationships with peers and teachers. Establish what the individual found rewarding and unrewarding about their educational experiences. Consider how the individual coped with any problems experienced within their educational environment.

3. *Occupational history.* Document what employment the individual has experienced. Problems might be evident with authority figures, such as employers or supervisors, and relationships with colleagues. If unemployed for significant periods, consider what may have accounted for this, for example, high unemployment rate, presence of significant mental or physical health problems, lack of interest in work.

4. *Relationship history.* Gather information on the individual's experience of intimate (romantic) relationships through adolescence and adulthood. In particular, pay attention to evidence of the ability to form and maintain close affective bonds. Consider areas of conflict within relationships and what strategies the individual has employed to resolve such conflicts. Establish how relationships have terminated. Where children have been involved, consider how well the individual has provided care, love and safety for the children.

5. *Psychiatric history.* Gather data pertaining to the individual's history of contact with mental health services. Consider the diagnoses offered and the relative success of intervention and management strategies. This may often provide essential information on how well an individual complies with attempts to provide support for mental health problems. Such a history may also point to unmet needs that might be crucial in establishing risk markers and identifying areas of work to attempt to reduce risk.

6. *Substance abuse history.* In particular, the relationship between substance abuse and violence should be established. For example, there may be important differences between violence that occurs to aid the acquisition of resources in order to support a dependency, and violence that may occur as a consequence of disinhibition or distress as a consequence of substance abuse. The impact of even moderate levels of substance abuse on mental and physical health should be considered. It is important here to document an individual's reasons for using substances and the various effects they may have had upon them, in addition to detailing what and how much the individual has used.

7. *Forensic history.* Document any previous arrests, charges and convictions. Where possible, establish any other additional information

about antisocial behaviour throughout the lifespan. Obtain and make reference to official documentation about offending behaviour. Consider any sentences deployed, the range of violent and non-violent offences perpetrated by the individual, and the response to any previous attempts to limit offending behaviour. In the UK data from the police national computer (PNC) system are usually made available during court hearings and these documents detail all offences associated with an individual. However, further information, such as witness statements, police interview transcripts and court-related documentation should also be sought, as these can provide valuable information that the individual may not recall or choose to disclose. In addition, there may be the need also to give some consideration to allegations made, particularly if these are numerous and from diverse sources.

A broad range of sources should be accessed in the compilation of this history. Self-report should not be solely relied upon, as individuals may simply be poor historians or motivated not to reveal certain aspects of their background. We all may have many reasons for hiding our shameful or hurtful experiences from others, as this offers protection from feelings of evaluation and judgement by them. Furthermore, some individuals may be disposed to attempt to deliberately deceive others in order to maximise their chances of liberty or opportunity to reoffend. Where possible, a range of relatives or close friends should be identified and accessed as additional sources of information. It is also wise to establish systems to access other sources that might corroborate or refute the data presented by the individual, such as general practitioner records, school reports, previous mental health service documentation and any other official sources that might be available.

Once an exhaustive history has been established, one of the actuarial measures should be applied. There are many such measures and the choice of which one may be baffling. However, some simple guidelines apply. First, ensure that the measure has been used before with individuals from a similar population to the person being assessed. Second, establish whether there is sufficient information available to complete the majority of the items, considering carefully how omitted items might affect the overall assessment. For example, in order to complete the sex offender risk appraisal guide fully, it may be necessary to conduct a penile plethysmograph assessment. This form of assessment in itself is problematic and there are typically scant appropriate resources available. Third, ensure that the target behaviour, such as violence, firesetting, sexual violence or general recidivism, is appropriately covered within the remit of the actuarial assessment. The skill of applying one of the actuarial measures does not lie in a minimalist approach. With each item, care should be taken to consider how much every factor applies to the individual and how this might be associated with their harmful behaviour.

Formulating risk

The above process leads naturally to the development of a formulation of risk of harmful behaviour. Here the risk factors, the potential harm and the probability of the behaviour recurring can be considered in detail. Moore (1996) offers a useful series of insights into the formulation of risk. Extending on the suggestions of Moore, we recommend the following considerations when constructing a formulation of risk.

1. It is important to establish the degree of error or bias that exists within the risk assessment. For example, there may be insufficient sources of information and it is key to consider how this has impacted on the assessment process. Other common errors are possible when compiling risk assessments. The appropriateness of any specific risk measures applied needs to be addressed. The use of invalid or unreliable instruments needs to be avoided. Have any false correlations been made that lead to causal interpretations, such as the relationship between schizophrenia and violence, or sex offending and recidivism? Here, the clinician will need to seek out the relevant base rates of behaviour. A good self-test is 'what percentage of people with schizophrenia kill?' and 'Of those that kill, what are the usual victim characteristics?' In response to this test, consider from where you may have derived any knowledgeable guesses. In summary, it is crucial to furnish the reader of any risk assessment with an understanding of the nature of any likely error and bias in the report. A simple statement can be added to conclusions to indicate whether there has been error leading to an overestimation or underestimation of bias.

2. Often risk assessment reports, particularly those featuring actuarial measures, fail to describe the target of the risk assessment adequately. Here, it is necessary to specify what harmful behaviour the individual is at risk of doing. For instance, there is likely to be a different mechanism for violence involved in the offender who assaults only their partner and the offender who only assaults strangers. If an individual has a history of specific forms of violence against different groups of victims, each of these will need to be defined. Only in this way can the risk formulation contribute to an explanation of the behaviour, rather than simply a generalised description.

3. In order to explain how and why an individual is judged to have a specific risk status, it is necessary to address the motivational drive of the individual and their previous use of violence. Some factors, such as mental illness or substance abuse, are too readily suggested as being the motivation for violent behaviour within a population of mentally disordered offenders. However, this rather naively assumes that the presence of mental illness and/or substance abuse is sufficient to explain why previous harmful behaviour occurred. In the most rudimentary terms, consider the potentially diverse motivations involved in the distress associated with the experience of mental illness leading to violence rather than the command of an omnipotent voice. The level of planning of harmful behaviour, the nature of the behaviour, the target of the behaviour and the individual emotional reaction may all differ greatly. Therefore, the function of the harmful behaviour needs to be considered, within the context of other

difficulties experienced by the individual. Clearly, this begins the process of planning for risk management. Take the example of a young man with schizophrenia who is violent to others under duress from an auditory hallucination. He may reluctantly strike out at those around him. The management of this individual will clearly involve engaging him in relationships where he feels comfortable to report the pressure he might experience from a voice, as medication alone is not guaranteed to be sufficient.

4. Harm-doing may be controlled by various factors, such as the empathy experienced for past victims, a moral code against the use of force and acknowledgement of the degree of risk posed. Similarly, it may be disinhibited by these factors or many others. Thus, when formulating the risk posed by an individual, it is essential to consider the presence or absence of controlling and disinhibiting factors. This permits a more dynamic understanding of the individual's current level of risk and allows for responsive flexibility in future management.

Consideration of the above leads the clinician through a process of formulating risk that goes towards developing a better understanding of the harmful behaviour. In turn, our experience has taught us how useful this process is in identifying specific risk markers for a given individual over and above the actuarial measures available.

IMPROVING MULTIDISCIPLINARY RISK ASSESSMENTS

No one individual can possibly acquire, let alone retain, all the information pertinent to risk assessment. Indeed, it is impossible to keep abreast of all new information that might relate to risk assessment. Hence, most of us gather and use information that relates to our interests or primary activities. Here, therefore, multidisciplinary working allows for a congregation of diverse understandings and explanations of harmful behaviour and the assessment of risk. The presentation of a risk assessment report or conclusions to a multidisciplinary meeting will naturally provoke some discussion about the veracity and utility of the conclusions drawn. Such discussion inevitably promotes objective scrutiny that can only enhance the risk assessment process. Multidisciplinary working, however, also readily improves the risk assessment process at numerous stages.

A multidisciplinary team should decide amongst its members a strategy for implementing risk assessment procedures. The first goal for the team is to decide how the risk assessment itself will be used and this goal can then be enshrined within policy documentation. The team will need to discuss whether they envisage actively operationalising the risk assessment. In other words, what is the completion of the risk assessment really likely to achieve? If the assessment is unlikely to contribute to ongoing management of individual clients of the team, then it would be futile to expend considerable effort on the completion of meaningful attempts at risk assessment. Alternatively, if the team feels that risk assessment is central to its ability to provide adequate care and support for an individual, then it will be important to complete as full a risk assessment as possible. Risk assessments for either purpose should establish a range of needs for the individual and the service providers.

For example, if someone's violence is mediated by their ongoing difficulties in intimate relationships, then appropriate support will have to be put in place to reduce the risk of harm. Clearly, any multidisciplinary team will need to consider the role and purpose of risk assessment carefully before selecting appropriate tools and methodologies.

Risk assessment is a blossoming field, and new measures and tools are frequently introduced. This provides for an ever-increasing range of needs to be met, with measures becoming more specific in the type of harmful behaviour they address. However, there can be a negative side to this within multidisciplinary working. Some professions are afforded more time for academic studies than others, which can mean that any new tools introduced will be owned by the few and not the many. This will inevitably be to the detriment of multidisciplinary risk assessment. Limiting the role of specific tools within the process can compensate for this, as all team members will remain expert in the process of risk assessment described here, such as reporting on historical factors and formulating risks. Furthermore, allowing a team to become expert in a specific tool that is broad enough to meet the needs of the majority of the population is likely to enhance multidisciplinary risk assessment. As experience of use increases, team members will grow in confidence about their ability to illuminate areas of risk assessment, becoming more mindful of what information would be helpful to the risk assessment process.

Applying a routine method for the compilation of risk assessments is intrinsic to good multidisciplinary functioning in this matter. A range of possibilities exists and the decision process about which to implement is aided by considering how the risk assessment will be used, what needs the individual being assessed might have, and the resources made available to the team for the completion of the task. For some teams, it might appeal to have one nominated member who takes an active lead of the risk assessment process. This person may then be involved in all the risk assessment reports or summaries prepared. This method has the advantage of crystallising expertise in risk assessment. However, there are some important disadvantages. If one person leads all the risk assessments, the opportunities for bias and error are increased, as other team members may feel unable to challenge or might see themselves as having no role in risk assessment. Thus, one person's perspective may have a dominant influence on the management of individuals. It follows that it is difficult for the team to own such an assessment.

A related problem lies in the nature by which information is gathered to inform the risk assessment process. If some team members are rarely involved in the risk assessment process, they may lose expertise in what information is important to aid the risk assessment. Thus, an individual talking about their attitudes during exercise or a social work meeting might have their opinions recorded differently than if they were discussing these issues with the person responsible for compiling the risk assessment process. An alternative method for risk assessment is to share responsibilities across people within the multidisciplinary team, with perhaps one individual taking responsibility for coordinating efforts.

Initially, this may delay individual learning and the overall realisation of quality assessments but has the useful function of firmly placing risk assessment on every team member's agenda. Furthermore, the shared expertise is likely to lead to more accurate risk assessments being produced (McNiel et al., 2000). The profile of professionals perhaps not typically involved in producing risk assessment reports can be developed by this means. By sharing the responsibility for preparing an assessment, individuals will learn the risk assessment process applied by the team. All clinicians within a multidisciplinary team can play a crucial role in gathering historical, present-day and future-related information. Ensuring, therefore, that all team members remain involved in the risk assessment process means that the accuracy and the predictive validity of the risk assessment can be enhanced.

We mentioned earlier that to compile a thorough risk assessment can take many hours. Consequently, all teams will be faced with concerns about the resources they make available to the risk assessment process. Where such assessments are considered an essential aspect of routine clinical practice, the time involved in compiling risk assessments is perhaps less important. However, ongoing training of all team members is necessary, which means that multidisciplinary teams will have to think carefully about how training budgets are to be used and allocated. One effective method is peer supervision and review. Regular reviews of reports by other team members or perhaps, confidentiality permitting, other teams, allows for regular quality assurance checks and may promote insight into areas of further training need. Other systems that work well may involve presentations related to conferences attended, the development of a risk assessment resource pack that all team members contribute to, including articles, good examples of anonymous reports and copies of any assessment tools, and regular review of the multidisciplinary team's risk assessment process, for example, documenting how the assessments are being used, considering the outcomes of the assessments and summarising the risk characteristics of the team's population so far.

Once the risk assessment has been completed, including an agreed formulation, the multidisciplinary team is then tasked with establishing when and who will update the risk assessment, in addition to developing a management strategy for the individual whose risk has been assessed. To facilitate this process, discussions can be had ahead of the risk assessment process to consider broadly how the team can respond to different global levels of risk. This typically leads to the development of strategy that documents what to do when an individual is categorised as high risk. For instance, most services would probably agree that high risk denotes the need for immediate intervention in a range of areas as specified by the risk assessment. Multidisciplinary working ideally allows for the demands of these processes to be shared. Similarly, the team can consider the development of standards of care associated with risk assessment, such as how long should someone identified as a moderate risk be subject to scrutiny? Many of these questions are usually answered within a good formulation of risk, but a broader level of discussion about team objectives can be helpful in clarifying difficult cases.

Finally, risk assessment is improved by multidisciplinary working primarily because of the strengths of teamwork. Responsibilities, tasks and expertise are shared, and all of these are key to effective risk assessment. Furthermore, the support available means that no one individual is likely to be stranded and unable to proceed with a difficult risk assessment. This process is summarized in Figure 8.1.

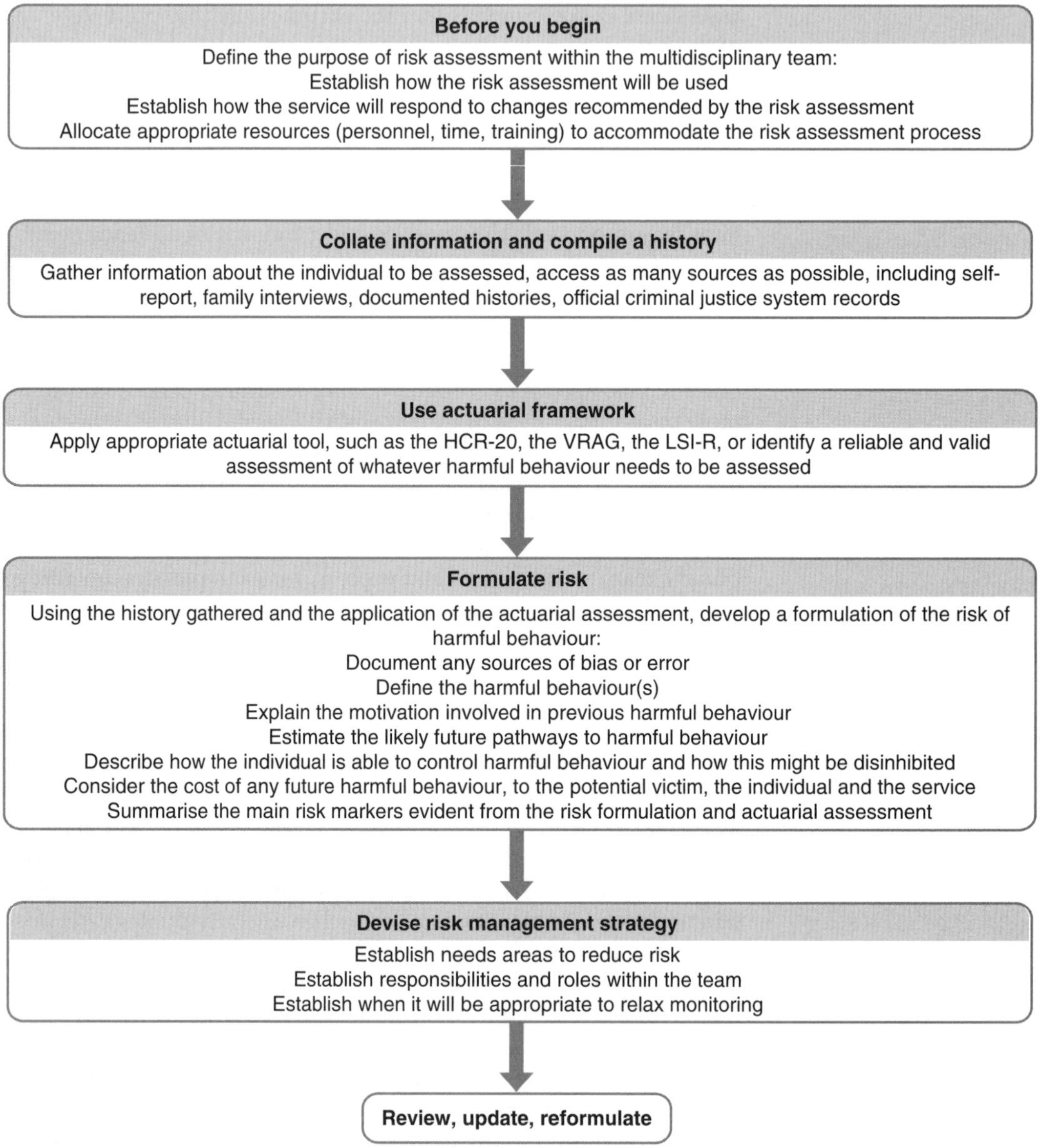

Before you begin
Define the purpose of risk assessment within the multidisciplinary team:
Establish how the risk assessment will be used
Establish how the service will respond to changes recommended by the risk assessment
Allocate appropriate resources (personnel, time, training) to accommodate the risk assessment process

Collate information and compile a history
Gather information about the individual to be assessed, access as many sources as possible, including self-report, family interviews, documented histories, official criminal justice system records

Use actuarial framework
Apply appropriate actuarial tool, such as the HCR-20, the VRAG, the LSI-R, or identify a reliable and valid assessment of whatever harmful behaviour needs to be assessed

Formulate risk
Using the history gathered and the application of the actuarial assessment, develop a formulation of the risk of harmful behaviour:
Document any sources of bias or error
Define the harmful behaviour(s)
Explain the motivation involved in previous harmful behaviour
Estimate the likely future pathways to harmful behaviour
Describe how the individual is able to control harmful behaviour and how this might be disinhibited
Consider the cost of any future harmful behaviour, to the potential victim, the individual and the service
Summarise the main risk markers evident from the risk formulation and actuarial assessment

Devise risk management strategy
Establish needs areas to reduce risk
Establish responsibilities and roles within the team
Establish when it will be appropriate to relax monitoring

Review, update, reformulate

Figure 8.1   Risk assessment process.

CONCLUDING REMARKS

The importance of risk assessment continues to be asserted at many levels within the health service and remains a central task within multidisciplinary working in mental health services. When multidisciplinary teams have been criticised in regard to risk assessment, this predominantly relates to issues of communication within and between teams (Appleby et al., 1999). The main aim of this summary of risk assessment has been to introduce a rationale for discussions within multidisciplinary teams about the process of risk assessment. A second aim has been to offer an update on available tools and recommended methods for compiling risk assessments that will promote the active management of risk problems by developing a good understanding and working formulation of an individual case.

References

Andrews D A (1982) The level of supervision inventory (LSI): The first follow-up. Toronto: Ontario Ministry of Correctional Services

Andrews D A and Bonta J L (1995) The level of service inventory-revised: user's manual. New York: Multi-Health Systems Inc

Appleby L, Shaw J, Amos T and McDonnell R (1999) Safer services: National Confidential Inquiry into suicide and homicide by people with mental illness. London: Department of Health

Blumenthal S and Lavender T (2000) Violence and mental disorder: a critical aid to the assessment and management of risk. London: Jessica Kingsely

Bonta J and Motiuk L L (1985) Utilization of an interview-based classification instrument: a study of correctional halfway houses. Criminal Justice and Behavior 12: 333–352

Doyle M, Dolan M and McGovern J (2002) The validity of North American risk assessment tools in predicting in-patient violent behaviour in England. Legal and Criminological Psychology 7: 141–154

Gray N S, McGleish A, MacCulloch M J, Hill C, Timmons D and Snowden R J (2003) Prediction of violence and self-harm in mentally disordered offenders: a prospective study of the efficacy of HCR-20, PCL-R, and psychiatric symptomatology. Journal of Consulting and Clinical Psychology 71: 443–451

Hare R D (1991) The Hare psychopathy checklist—revised: manual. Toronto: Multi-Health Systems, Inc

Hare R D (1993) Without conscience: the disturbing world of psychopaths among us. New York: The Guilford Press

Heilbrun K (1997) Prediction vs. management models relevant to risk assessment: the importance of legal decision-making context. Law and Human Behavior 21: 347–359

Hemphill J F, Hare R D and Wong S (1998) Psychopathy and recidivism: a review. Legal and Criminological Psychology 3: 139–170

Howlett M (1998) Medication, non-compliance and mentally disordered offenders. London: The Zito Trust

Kraemer H C, Kazdin A E, Offord D R, Kessler R C, Jensen P S and Kupfer D J (1997) Coming to terms with the terms of risk. Archives of General Psychiatry 54: 337–343

Lidz C W, Mulvey E P and Gardner W A (1993) The accuracy of predictions of violence to others. JAMA: Journal of the American Medical Association 8: 1007–1011

Link B G and Stueve A (1994) Evidence bearing on mental illness as a possible cause of violent behaviour. Epidemiological Reviews 17: 172–181

Martell D A, Rosner R and Harmon R B (1995) Base-rate estimates of criminal behaviour by homeless mentally ill persons in New York City. Psychiatric Services 46: 596–601

McNeil D E (1994) Hallucinations and violence. In: Monahan J and Steadman H (eds) Violence and mental disorder: developments in risk assessment. Chicago: Chicago University Press

McNeil D E, Lam J N and Binder R L (2000) Relevance of interrater agreement to violence risk assessment. Journal of Consulting and Clinical Psychology 68: 1111–1115

Modestin J and Ammann R (1995) Mental disorders and criminal behaviour. British Journal of Psychiatry 166: 667–675

Monahan J (1992) Mental disorder and violent behaviour: perceptions and evidence. American Psychologist 47: 511–521

Monahan J (1993) Causes of violence. In: USS Commission (ed.) Drugs and violence in America. Washington, DC: US Government Printing Office

Monahan J and Steadman H (1994) Toward a rejuvenation of risk assessment research. In: Monahan J and Steadman H (eds) Violence and mental disorder: developments in risk assessment. Chicago: Chicago University Press

Monahan J, Steadman H J, Silver E, Appelbaum P S, Clark Robbins P, Mulvey E P, Roth LH, Grisso T and Banks S (2001) Rethinking risk assessment: the MacArthur study of mental disorder and violence. Oxford: Oxford University Press

Moore B (1996) Risk assessment: a practitioners guide to predicting harmful behaviour. London: Whiting and Birch

Quinsey V L, Harris G T, Rice M E and Cormier C A (1998) Violent offenders: appraising and managing risk. Washington, DC: American Psychological Association

Rice M E and Harris G T (1997) The treatment of mentally disordered offenders. Psychology, Public Policy and Law 3: 126–183

Royal College of Psychiatrists (1998) Management of imminent violence: clinical practice guidelines to support mental health services. Occasional paper OP41. London: Royal College of Psychiatry College Research Unit

Silver E, Mulvey E P and Monahan J (1999) Assessing violence risk among discharged psychiatric patients: towards an ecological approach. Law and Human Behaviour 23: 237–255

Singleton N, Meltzer H, Gatward R, Coid J and Deasy D (1998) Psychiatric morbidity among prisoners. London: Stationary Office

Steadman H J, Monahan J, Robbins P C, Appelbaum P, Grisso T, Klassen D, Mulvey E P and Roth L (1993) From dangerousness to risk assessment: implications for appropriate research strategies. In: Hodgins S (ed.) Mental disorder and crime. Newbury Park, CA: Sage Publications

Steadman H J, Mulvey E P, Monahan J, Robbins P C, Appelbaum P S, Grisso T, Roth L H and Silver E (1998) Violence by people discharged from acute psychiatric inpatient facilities and by others in the same neighbourhoods. Archives of General Psychiatry 55: 1–9

Swanson J, Holzer C, Gunju V and Jono R (1990) Violence and psychiatric disorder in the community: evidence from the epidemiological catchments area surveys. Hospital and Community Psychiatry 41: 761–770

Swartz M S, Swanson J W, Hiday V A, Borum R, Wagner H R and Burns B J (1998) Violence and severe mental illness: the effects of substance abuse and non-adherence to medication. American Journal of Psychiatry 155: 226–231

Tennent T G (1975) The dangerous offender. In: Barraclough B and Silverstone T (eds) Contemporary psychiatry. Ashford: Headley Brothers

Thomas-Peter B A and Jones J P (2004) High risk inferences in assessing high risk: outstanding concerns in the clinical use of the PCL-R. Journal of Forensic Psychiatry and Psychology (in press)

Webster C D, Douglas K S, Eaves D and Hart S D (1997) HCR-20: Assessing risk of violence (version 2). Vancouver: Mental Health Law and Policy Institute, Simon Fraser University

Chapter **9**

Treatment planning, medication management and the forensic multidisciplinary team

Deborah Robson, Stuart Wix and Richard Gray

INTRODUCTION

Forensic mental health services provide care and treatment to people suffering from a range of disorders. Effective, collaborative, treatment planning and good medication management represent a very real challenge in a forensic environment. Increasingly, modern health care is driven by consumer choice and empowerment. Good medication management practice is about helping service users get the most out of this component of their treatment by making informed treatment decisions. Our aim in this chapter is to discuss effective treatment planning and medication management in a forensic context.

POLICY

The National Institute for Clinical Excellence (NICE) has produced two documents that are important in medication management that mental health care professionals need to take into account when exercising their clinical judgement. The first was an appraisal of the use of antipsychotics in the treatment of schizophrenia (NICE, 2002), and the second, clinical guidelines on core interventions in the same illness (NICE, 2003). These build on parts of the National Service Framework for mental health (Department of Health, 1999) and are intended to inform the evolution of service development plans. Local health communities are expected to review existing service provision against the standards identified. It is hoped that the guidelines will enhance the care that patients receive by improving the quality of clinical decision-making. More information about the NICE schizophrenia guidelines is available at www.nice.org.uk.

Effective treatment of mental illness relies upon a clearly formulated and defined package of multidisciplinary care involving all the various available forms of appropriate assessment, intervention and treatment, including pharmacological and psychosocial approaches. The planning, management and evaluation of the use of prescribed medicines within mental health services has, traditionally, been the domain of psychiatrists, with nurses and pharmacists playing a supporting role. With the policy implementation of extended and supplementary prescribing for both mental health nurses and pharmacists now a reality, and discussions taking place regarding clinical psychologists being given prescribing powers, these tasks can now be shared amongst members of the multidisciplinary team, possibly giving more choice to the patient. Medication management, using psychosocial interventions, such as compliance therapy (Kemp et al., 1998), is now very much a multidisciplinary responsibility rather than being the preserve of doctors and nurses.

THE PRACTICE OF MULTIDISCIPLINARY TREATMENT PLANNING

Some of the patients who are the most disturbed and difficult to engage and treat in the entire field of mental health are often managed in forensic settings. It is, therefore, crucial that treatment decision-making, assessment, review of treatment effectiveness and evaluation are founded upon sound collaborative, multidisciplinary team working. As already stated, the role of the prescriber within teams is set to change in the near future with a shift toward collaborative or supplementary prescribing, with partnerships between psychiatrists and nurses, or psychiatrists and pharmacists likely to become the norm. However, at present, the existing model of treatment planning and prescribing in forensic mental health care remains the domain of medicine, with psychiatrists taking a leading role.

Traditionally, wide ranges of professional disciplines contribute to the multidisciplinary process of treatment planning, with a core group of professionals adopting a more proactive role. Whilst most professional team members can comment on the wider observed effects of physical treatment on a patient, be it the recognition of side effects or the reporting of symptom reduction, key disciplines can play a more considered and critical role. The function and presence of a clinical pharmacist as part of a multidisciplinary team, for example, cannot be underestimated. As already implied in Chapter 3, a clinical pharmacist may, in many instances, enhance treatment decision-making, for instance, through the preparation and discussion of a detailed drug history for individual patients, which can assist a team to examine the effectiveness of previous treatment strategies. The clinical pharmacist may also provide additional clinical advice to the multidisciplinary team with regard to the safest, most rational and economic use of pharmacological treatment.

A range of disciplines within the context of the multidisciplinary team working may contribute to the process of treatment planning by utilising a range of assessment tools to assess the effectiveness of drug treatment over time, for example, by the use of the KGV-M (Krawiecka Goldberg Vaughn—Modified) rating scale or in determining the presence of side effects (e.g. by application of the Liverpool University Neuroleptic Side Effect Rating Scale). Various members of the team may be able to establish the patient's view and beliefs about treatment, for example, by use of the Hogan Drug Attitude Inventory (Hogan et al., 1983).

The regime of treatment prescribed can also be closely monitored and reviewed regularly, in collaboration with the patient, to maximise adherence. Polypharmacy should be avoided, where one change at a time to the treatment regime will be the norm to prevent a confused picture (Barkley, 2000). NICE guidelines (2002: 10), for example, recommend 'It is best to use a single drug, using doses within the British National Formulary (BNF) dose range and not to use high or loading doses'.

Given that a sizeable proportion of forensic psychiatric patients have a chronic and enduring mental illness, the use of a detailed drug history can prove invaluable, particularly when clinicians are seeking to achieve the ideal of avoiding polypharmacy and devising treatment plans that are uncomplicated. It is also important to stress that the best outcomes for patients with regard to symptom reduction, side-effect management and treatment adherence is likely to be achieved through a process of effective collaboration, where treatment planning is devised, managed or monitored by suitably trained, experienced and motivated professionals.

GUIDANCE ON THE USE OF ATYPICAL ANTIPSYCHOTICS

Based on the current available evidence, NICE (2002) have recommended the following clinical practice guidelines on the use of atypical antipsychotics. These relate to good multidisciplinary practice.

- The choice of drug should be made jointly between the individual and the clinician involving the carer, if appropriate.
- Atypical antipsychotics should be the first-line treatment for schizophrenia.
- Individuals on typical antipsychotics should be considered for atypical drugs, if they experience unpleasant side effects.
- Clozapine is the treatment of choice for treatment-resistant schizophrenia.
- Clinicians should undertake an adherence assessment. If there is a risk of users not taking their medication, then a long-acting formulation should be considered.
- Antipsychotic medication is part of a comprehensive package of care.
- Atypical and typical antipsychotics should not be prescribed at the same time.

CORE INTERVENTIONS IN THE TREATMENT AND MANAGEMENT OF SCHIZOPHRENIA IN PRIMARY AND SECONDARY CARE

Guidelines on core interventions in the treatment and management of schizophrenia were published in 2003 (NICE, 2003). The guidance reiterates much of what was set out in the technology appraisal on the use of anti-psychotics, with some additions. The key points are listed below.

- Principles of treatment:
  - Assessment and care planning should be collaborative, positive, optimistic and should be delivered within a multidisciplinary context.
  - Information shared with users and carers should be clear and understandable.
  - Service users should state their preferences for treatment choices in the event of an acute episode. Where consultation is not possible, an atypical antipsychotic should be the first choice.
- Treatment in the acute episode: pharmacological interventions:
  - The minimum effective dose should be used.
  - Atypicals and typicals should not be prescribed at the same time.
  - Regular screening, monitoring and management of the side effects of medication including extrapyramidal symptoms (dystonia, akathisia, parkinsonian), and cholinergic, sexual, cardiac and endocrinological side effects.
- Promoting recovery:
  - Both service users and carers should be given the opportunity to tell their own stories about their illness history and experiences of treatment, and have it recorded in their case notes.
  - Services users should be asked about their satisfaction with their prescribed medicines.
  - Cognitive behavioural therapy is recommended to develop users insight and promote treatment adherence.
  - Following an acute episode, treatment should continue for 1–2 years. Stopping antipsychotic medication should be gradual.
  - Once medication has stopped, the service user should be followed up for 2 years.
  - Clozapine should be considered at the earliest opportunity for those users who have not responded to two antipsychotics within a 6–8 week period (including one atypical).
  - A depot antipsychotic should be considered where:
    - medication avoidance is a problem;
    - a user chooses or finds a depot more convenient.

INTERPRETATION OF THESE GUIDELINES IN A FORENSIC POPULATION

Most of the recent policy documents have focused on the care and treatment of people with schizophrenia. The NICE (2003) schizophrenia guidelines specifically state that they do not apply to people with the illness who have a very early or very late onset, who have a coexisting learning difficulty; a coexisting substance use problem; physical or sensory difficulties or who are homeless. Most people who use forensic services fall into one or other of these latter groups. In addition, there are special considerations relating to compliance in a forensic population where relapse may be linked directly with increased risk to the individual or others, the possibility of further offending, or disturbed dangerous behaviour. Depot antipsychotic preparations, by their very nature, therefore, may have a particular place in the treatment of certain patients or groups of patients. This is likely to be the case especially where there is uncertainty about the degree of insight the individual concerned might have.

HOW EFFECTIVE ARE DRUG TREATMENTS FOR MENTAL DISORDER?

Much of the evidence about the effectiveness of psychotropic medication comes from trials conducted in unrepresentative populations of service users. People who consent to take part in drug trials are certainly not representative of a forensic population. Nevertheless, this is the best evidence that is currently available and may be used to inform clinical practice. A variety of drugs are used in forensic environments including antipsychotics; antidepressants; mood stabilisers; anxiolytics and hypnotics. In addition, there are those used in the emergency situation for so-called rapid tranquillisation.

ANTIPSYCHOTICS

Antipsychotic medication has been the mainstay of treatment for schizophrenia since the 1950s when it was discovered that the dopamine antagonists, haloperidol and chlorpromazine, exerted antipsychotic effects.

Chlorpromazine, the first effective pharmacological treatment for the symptoms of schizophrenia, was introduced during the 1950s. Since then, a variety of antipsychotic agents have been developed, some of which are available in a long-acting depot formulation. Controlled clinical trials have repeatedly shown that these drugs are generally efficacious for treatment of the positive symptoms of schizophrenia. About eight out of ten users can expect to gain some benefit from treatment, with about a 50% reduction in positive symptoms, such as hallucinations and delusions. However, these medicines may make some negative symptoms for instance self-isolation and withdrawal worse. Tolerability problems, especially to do with acute extrapyramidal effects (EPS), dystonias, akathisia and Parkinsonism, are relatively common with these conventional agents.

Conventional antipsychotics are also associated with a range of other common side effects, including sexual and reproductive dysfunction, and anticholinergic symptoms that include dry mouth, blurred vision and constipation, as well as sedation and weight gain. Antipsychotics can also cause the rare but potentially fatal idiosyncratic dose-independent reaction of neuroleptic malignant syndrome (NMS). The main symptoms are hyperthermia or fever and severe muscle rigidity. The incidence is unknown but may occur in up to 0.15% of people treated with antipsychotics.

Many people who take antipsychotic medication are concerned about the long-term effects. It is known that antipsychotics can cause tardive dyskinesia. It is generally thought that 5% of people treated with typical antipsychotics will develop these symptoms with each year of exposure to the medicine. Tardive dyskinesia, especially when more severe, will make people stand out and contributes to the stigma of mental illness generally and schizophrenia specifically.

THE NEED FOR NEW TREATMENTS

The unacceptable side-effect profile of antipsychotic medicines and a lack of efficacy in treating negative symptoms have prompted further research into the development of improved novel and atypical agents, such as clozapine, risperidone, olanzapine and quetiapine. Atypical antipsychotics cause fewer EPS, in fact, they are no more likely than a placebo drug to do so. However, that is not to say that they are free from side effects. One atypical antipsychotic was voluntarily withdrawn by its manufacturers in 1998 because of concerns over cardiac safety (Gray, 2001b).

A reduction in side effects is not the only difference between typical and atypical antipsychotics. When the data from a large number of clinical trials are pooled together, it is clear that risperidone, olanzapine and quetiapine (Gray, 2001a) are effective treatments for schizophrenia producing clinically meaningful improvements in symptoms and preventing relapse. However, they are no more effective at doing this than conventional antipsychotics, such as chlorpromazine or haloperidol. Clozapine shows that uniquely it is more effective than typical antipsychotics but is not widely used because of its side-effect profile. There is emerging evidence that atypical antipsychotics may also be effective in treating negative symptoms. There is also interesting preliminary work suggesting that atypicals may also be useful in treating cognitive symptoms, reducing violence and aggression, suicidality, craving for illicit substances and alcohol and, perhaps most importantly, improving users' health-related quality of life (Gray, 2001a).

Implications for clinical practice

- Antipsychotics are effective in reducing psychotic symptoms for many service users.
- Atypical antipsychotics generally cause fewer side effects than conventional treatments.
- Atypical antipsychotics may offer additional therapeutic benefits over traditional treatments.

ANTIDEPRESSANTS

From a biological perspective, it has been proposed that depression is caused by a reduction in either serotonin or noradrenaline (norepinephrine), and mania by an excess of noradrenaline. Tricyclic antidepressants (TCAs) and selective serotonin reuptake inhibitors (SSRIs) prevent the reuptake of these neurotransmitters at the pre-synaptic neurone. This mechanism increases the amount of neurotransmitter at the synapse. Over the past decade, the use of TCAs in both primary and secondary care settings has reduced dramatically. TCAs have now been largely replaced by SSRIs and other novel antidepressants, such as venlafaxine. SSRIs do not cause many of the side effects associated with traditional TCAs and are safer in overdose. The main side effects associated with SSRIs are nausea and agitation. They have also been associated with sexual dysfunction in both men and women and, less commonly, dry mouth and sedation.

Implications for clinical practice

- Antidepressants are effective in the treatment of depression.
- SSRIs are safer and generally better tolerated than TCAs.

MOOD STABILISERS

Mood stabilisers are widely used to treat bipolar affective disorder and other related conditions, such as unipolar depression and schizoaffective disorder. There is also evidence that lithium is effective in treating some non-affective mental health problems, such as borderline personality disorder. Lithium has been the front-line drug for bipolar disorder for many years, although increasingly carbamazepine and sodium valporate are becoming more popular.

Implications for clinical practice

- Lithium is an effective mood stabiliser but requires close monitoring.
- Carbamazepine and sodium valporate are also well-tolerated and effective mood stabilisers.

ANTIANXIETY AND SEDATIVE–HYPNOTIC DRUGS

Benzodiazepines are the most widely prescribed group of drugs in the world, although in recent years, their popularity has waned because of their potential to cause tolerance and dependence. Benzodiazepines have a wide range of uses, including in anxiety, anxiety-related phobias, alcohol withdrawal and sleep disorders. They may also be used in the treatment of acute agitation and aggression. Prolonged use can result in physical dependency. Withdrawal symptoms range from insomnia and anxiety to extreme agitation and convulsions, and may be fatal, if not treated appropriately. However, if prescribed, short-term dependence can be avoided, especially if treatment is stopped gradually. It is also useful to advise service users to use benzodiazepines intermittently rather than regularly to reduce the risk of tolerance and dependence.

The use of barbiturates has largely been replaced by benzodiazepines as antianxiety and sedative–hypnotic drugs because of tolerability and safety issues. Two drugs that are not structurally related to benzodiazepines and are licensed for the treatment of insomnia are zopiclone and zolpidem. Other drugs that may be useful antianxiety and sedative–hypnotic drugs include some antihistamines, propranolol and buspirone.

Implications for clinical practice

- Benzodiazepines are useful in the short-term treatment of anxiety, as well as alcohol withdrawal and sleep disorders.
- They may also be used in the treatment of acute agitation and aggression in patients with psychosis.
- They can lead to dependence if not closely monitored.

EMERGENCY TREATMENT

The use of medication to control disturbed behaviour by so-called 'rapid tranquillisation' (RT) is often seen as a last resort when other forms of intervention have failed or are considered inappropriate. The aim of RT is to calm the service user, and reduce the risk of violence and harm. The benefits of these approaches have to be balanced against the potential for medication to cause unwanted adverse effects. Although the evidence is limited, studies suggest that RT is a generally safe procedure (Pilowsky et al., 1992). However, the adverse events that have been reported following RT have been potentially serious cardiovascular and cardiorespiratory events (Pilowsky et al., 1992). Acute EPS may also be seen following the administration of medication by an intramuscular injection. These symptoms can be distressing to users and, in the case of akathisia and dystonia, may exacerbate disturbed behaviour. RT is a joint medical and nursing intervention. Good practice involves offering oral medication prior to considering the use of the intramuscular route of administration, regular monitoring of vital signs and the use of anticholinergic medication where necessary. There are guidelines available on the use of RT (Taylor et al., 2003).

THE NEED FOR MAINTENANCE TREATMENT

Some service users with mental illness will need to take medication continuously to prevent symptoms returning (Marder, 1999; Gray, 2001). Professionals describe people who stop taking medication as 'non-compliant'. Non-compliance infers a power imbalance where a passive 'patient' has not done what an 'expert', be it doctor, nurse or other professional, has told them to do. As the NICE guidelines suggest, modern health care is about partnership and collaboration. For many, the use of language, such as 'compliance' is unacceptable. Concordance may be a better term, as it suggests a collaborative process of decision-making regarding treatment (Gray et al., 2002). However, changing language alone will not change health care professionals' practice.

It is common for patients to stop antipsychotic medication. Although estimates vary, it seems likely that about 50% of service users who begin treatment with antipsychotic medication will have stopped taking it within a year of starting and that 75% will stop within 2 years (Weiden and Olfson, 1995). Virtually all of those who stop medication will experience a worsening of their psychosis or a relapse that may require hospitalisation. Such high rates may initially seem alarming. However, they are surprisingly similar to those seen, not only with other psychotropic medication, but also in other conditions, such as hypertension, human immunodeficiency virus (HIV), diabetes or asthma where maintenance treatment is required. Deviating from prescribed treatment is not uncommon or unusual, and should be thought of as normal behaviour. Stopping antipsychotic medication can be extremely concerning in a forensic setting, however, where relapse can result in the potential risk of harm to others.

WHY DON'T PEOPLE TAKE THEIR MEDICATION?

There appear to be a large number of factors that influence people's decisions about taking medication (Gray et al., 2002). These are summarised in Table 9.1. The common theme that emerges from the evidence

Table 9.1 Factors that influence service users' decisions about taking medication

Less likely to take medication	More likely to take medication
Side effects	Acceptance of illness
Negative beliefs about treatment	Perception of severity/susceptibility
Lack of perceived benefit	Level of support
Complex treatment regime	Family stability
Substance use	Positive therapeutic alliance
Impaired judgement	Route of administration
Poor clinician–service user relationship	Simple treatment regime
Poor communication between service user and multidisciplinary team	

is that the way in which people make decisions about whether or not to take medication is complex. Interventions, therefore, need to address the particular concerns that people have about taking medication and should be seen as a multidisciplinary responsibility and task.

EFFECTIVE INTERVENTIONS

Much of the research that has been conducted on interventions to help people to be better at taking psychotropic medication has evaluated the impact of service user education. Educational interventions aim to provide information to patients about both their illness and medication, with the goal of increasing understanding and promoting adherence. Service-user education has been evaluated using a variety of methodologies, including a number of randomised controlled trials (Macpherson et al., 1996; Gray, 2000). Results of these studies have shown that just giving information will improve service users' understanding of their illness and their medication, but will not reduce the numbers who stop taking medication. This is perhaps not surprising, given that educational interventions fail to address many of the important factors that influence people's decisions about taking medication.

In recent years, research into improving the taking of medication has focused on approaches based on cognitive behavioural therapy and motivational interviewing (Gray et al., 2002). Kemp et al. (1998) devised compliance therapy based on these techniques. The key principles of this approach include working collaboratively with service users, emphasising personal choice and responsibility and focusing on concerns about treatment. The intervention is divided into three phases. Phase 1 deals with service users' experiences of treatment by helping them review their illness history. In phase 2, common concerns about treatment are discussed, and the not so good and the good aspects about treatment are explored. Phase 3 deals with long-term prevention and strategies for avoiding relapse. Compliance therapy has been evaluated in a randomised controlled trial (Kemp et al., 1998). Seventy-four service users were randomly assigned to receive either compliance therapy or non-specific counselling. They received 4–6 sessions with a research psychiatrist lasting, on average, 40 minutes. When they were followed up 18 months after the start of the study, fewer relapses were seen in those who had received compliance therapy.

Implications for clinical practice

Psychiatric medication is effective and useful. However, many service users derive relatively limited benefit from treatment and many experience unwanted side effects. Poor adherence is also clearly a major problem, especially in forensic environments. Careful multidisciplinary treatment planning and good medication management will ensure that service users get the most out of taking their medication.

In treatment planning and medication management, good practice involves:

- A collaborative positive approach to working with users where arguing is avoided.
- A careful assessment of the positive and negative effects of medication.
- The user's views of medication.
- The user's understanding of medication.
- User's and carers' experiences of their illness and treatment.
- Exchanging information with service users about their problems, treatment options and goals.
- Multidisciplinary medication review and tailoring medication regimes to suit the service user, for example, the time of medication, dose, formulation.
- Using motivational interviewing to explore user's past experience of treatments and any ambivalence about taking medication.
- The use of cognitive behavioural techniques to address beliefs and views about medication.

The remainder of this chapter describes some practical clinical skills that the mental health worker may find helpful in translating the above recommendations into clinical practice.

ENGAGEMENT

The tension between ensuring that patients take medication as advised, but also maintaining a collaborative, user-centred approach and promoting choice is particularly pronounced in forensic settings. In order to reduce this, it is essential that we pay attention to the engagement process, not only viewing this as something we do at the beginning of our contact with users but something that we should work on throughout the therapeutic relationship. Part of the engagement process is about defining the areas where care and treatment is statutory and imposed, and that which is voluntary. This part of a forensic worker's role may cause antagonism with the user and cause the user to be resistant to talking about medication. Resistance can be reduced and engagement improved by making the whole process transparent and being consistent in approach. It is helpful to plan and structure each session depending on the user's level of functioning. At the beginning of each session, the patient, carer and worker should set an agenda with specific areas identified for discussion and considered achievable for the time allowed. Additional general therapeutic techniques that help keep people engaged include warmth of approach, displaying therapeutic optimism, checking that the patient understands what is being said and that the worker understands what they are saying, summarising, helping explore problems and assisting the service user to draw their own conclusions, and asking for feedback about how the session has gone.

ASSESSMENT

Traditionally, different professional groups have their own assessment 'language'. Working in a forensic multidisciplinary team requires all those concerned to possess generic assessment and treatment abilities in addition to their own professional skills. There are a number of reasons why assessment is a key component to good multidisciplinary medication treatment planning. Assessments can provide much more than diagnostic information. They are useful in detecting, measuring and monitoring symptoms, side effects, positive effects and adherence, which then informs the collaborative planning of care between the service user, carer and multidisciplinary team. The valid and accurate measurement of the response to a planned intervention is essential and is a requirement for all service users and carers, and not simply done for the sake of collecting data. People should be presented with a rationale for each assessment and given a copy of the summary of the assessment, if they wish to have one.

There is a range of assessment tools that can be used as part of good medication management. These include the following.

Assessing psychopathology

KGV-M (Lancashire, 1998)

In order to assess and evaluate the effectiveness of medicines, there are a number of reliable and valid rating scales that the forensic mental health worker can use. The KGV-M is made up of 13 symptom scales and a rating for the accuracy of the assessment. Its purpose is to elicit and measure the severity of psychotic symptoms in the month prior to interview. Ratings for anxiety, depressed mood, elevated mood, suicidal thoughts, delusions and hallucinations are based on the verbal report of the user. Ratings for flattened affect, incongruous affect, overactivity, psychomotor retardation, abnormal speech, poverty of speech and abnormal movements are based on the observation of the user's behaviour during the interview. The measure is only reliable when used by an appropriately trained and experienced rater (Lancashire, 1998).

Assessing side effects

Liverpool University Neuroleptic Side Effect Rating Scale (LUNSERS; Day et al., 1995)

Perhaps the most widely used measure of antipsychotic side effects is the LUNSERS, a 51-item self-report measure. Forty-one items, covering psychological, neurological, autonomic, hormonal and miscellaneous side effects, were constructed by rephrasing items from the UKU adverse events measure (Lingjaerde et al., 1987), so that they could be self-rated. The remaining ten items were 'red herrings' referring to symptoms, which were not known antipsychotic side effects (e.g. chilblains). Each item is rated on a five-point scale ranging from 'not at all' to 'very much' based on how frequently the patient has experienced the side effect in the last month. The LUNSERS is an efficient, reliable and valid method of monitoring antipsychotic side effects. Day et al. (1995) showed good test–retest reliability and concurrent validity against the UKU. It has also been demonstrated that there is a significant but weak correlation between increasing doses of antipsychotic medication and the number and frequency of side effects measured using the LUNSERS (Day et al., 1995).

Barnes Akathisia Rating Scale (BARS; Barnes, 1989)

The BARS is probably the most widely used measure of drug-induced akathisia. It is divided into three sections. An objective rating is scored from 0–3, that is, the user has normal to constant movement of the limbs. The second is a subjective rating where the patient rates how much they are aware of their restlessness and how distressed they are by it. Finally, the worker gives a global rating of the severity of the akathisia. The BARS has good validity and reliability.

Abnormal Involuntary Movement Scale (AIMS; Guy, 1976)

The AIMS is a 12-item scale that assesses abnormal involuntary movements commonly associated with typical antipsychotic medicines, such as tardive dyskinesia and akathisia, and has established inter-rater reliability. Scoring the AIMS consists of rating the service user's body movements in three main areas, namely facial and oral, extremities and trunk, each on a five-point scale. It also provides a global rating of severity, incapacitation and the patient's subjective awareness of the movements.

Assessing beliefs about treatment

The Hogan Drug Attitude Inventory (DAI-30; Hogan et al., 1983)

The DAI is a 30-item self-report measure predictive of compliance in people with schizophrenia. Each statement is rated as being true or false. The measure produces a total score ranging from +30 to −30. A positive score is predictive of compliance, a negative score of non-compliance. The scale has been shown to have a degree of discriminative validity, with 99% agreement between the DAI and clinical rating of whether patients were compliant or non-compliant.

Insight

Insight Scale (IS; Birchwood et al.,1994)

Scales to assess insight are problematic, as they can be complex to use in clinical practice. The Insight Scale is a self-report instrument that consists of eight statements (four negative, four positive). Patients can agree, disagree or be unsure. Questions include those around the need for medication, illness recognition and relabelling psychotic experiences.

Assessing practical issues

It is often taken for granted that patients know what they are prescribed and why they are prescribed it. It is, nevertheless, important to identify the service user's understanding of what medicines they are currently taking, the dose and frequency, and their understanding of why it has been prescribed. The practical arrangements for the prescription, supply and administration of medicines also need to be identified.

Rating importance, confidence and satisfaction about medication

It can also be useful to ask the service user to rate on a scale of 1–10:

- How important do you think it is to take your prescribed medication?
- How confident are you in taking your prescribed medication?
- How satisfied are you with your prescribed medication?

PLANNING

The outcome of all these potential assessments will provide a wealth of information but this is only useful if it informs the planning stage of the multidisciplinary approach to medication management. Any goals set should reflect any problems the patient might have identified, and should aim to be realistic, achievable, measurable and ideally recorded in their own words.

INTERVENTIONS

A variety of interventions can be used to help service users and carers get the most out of taking their medication.

Exchanging information

Opportunities should be taken to check the user's understanding of their treatment throughout and at each point of contact. This may begin with the exchange of information by asking the service user and carer what they already know about the illness and medicines they are taking. More information can then be offered with a clear and unambiguous explanation. Verbal information should be supported with written information and there should be a check that this has been understood. Information exchange is not a one-off event and should be an ongoing process.

Sorting out practical problems

If any practical problems have been identified in the assessment stage, such as difficulty in obtaining prescriptions, these need to be remedied using a problem-solving approach before moving on. It is more empowering for the user if they are central to the problem-solving process. Any difficulties identified can be worked through using a cognitive behavioural approach. The user then describes their problem and the desired goal in their own words. They are then encouraged to think about all the possible solutions to the problem. The user then writes down the good and not so good things about each solution. He or she then chooses what they think might be the best solution and identifies broad steps they need to take to put the solution into action. A date is then set to review the action plan.

Looking back

As recommended in the guidelines for core interventions for schizophrenia (NICE, 2003), service users and carers should be given the opportunity to tell the stories of their experiences of illness and treatment. This may be beneficial in identifying what treatment strategies in the past have worked well, and those that have not worked so well or have been perceived as such and are, therefore, likely to prove potentially problematic in the future. This may help develop awareness for the patient of the importance of taking medication to maintain health. However, it is important to bear in mind that, by looking back over repeated failures, users' confidence might equally be undermined.

Talking about negative treatment experiences

Asking users and carers to look back over their history of treatment may often uncover negative experiences of mental health care. For example, people may have very unpleasant memories of being restrained and given medication by intramuscular injection. Carers may have stories to tell about the difficulties in getting their relative to see a doctor for the first time or access to services as a whole. These experiences should not be ignored. The mental health worker should acknowledge and explore them where possible, and discuss how the user or carer can be more involved in, and feel more in control of, future treatment decisions.

Exploring ambivalence

Where users and carers have a variety of beliefs about treatment and are uncertain about the importance of taking medication, it may be helpful to examine the not so good and good things about taking medication, as well as the good and the not so good things about stopping medication. Experience seems to suggest that the majority of people have a degree of ambivalence about taking medication and, therefore, this is an exercise that should be done with every user. There may also be a distinction between short- and long-term benefits of taking medication. The aim is to help the user to explore their personal reasons for taking or not taking medication. As such, it is not rigid and rational like an accountant's balance sheet, but is often riddled with unique perceptions and idiosyncrasies. This approach can also be used to explore the good things and not so good things about using illegal substances, and the not so good things and good things about reducing or stopping their use.

Identifying the less obvious benefits of medication

Where patients fail to see any link between taking medication and symptom reduction, it may be useful to spend some time identifying the less obvious benefits of taking medication (e.g. staying out of hospital, not getting into arguments or fights, getting on better with other family members). Asking users about how things were when they were not taking medication compared with how things are now best does this. It may also be helpful to ask the user how family and friends view their medication. Identifying these less obvious benefits may increase the perceived importance of taking medication by increasing the personal relevance.

Talking about beliefs about illness and medication

From the Drug Attitude Inventory (Hogan et al., 1983) and having completed several sessions with the user, a formulation about the users' beliefs about their illness and treatment should have emerged. Often these beliefs will affect the importance users place on taking medication, for example, the belief that medication can be stopped when the service user feels better or that medication is addictive. In addition to providing accurate information, the patient can be helped to explore their beliefs so that they can draw their own conclusions. Such beliefs should be discussed one at a time. Users can be asked to rate how convinced they are that their belief is accurate on a percentage scale (0%, which is not accurate at all, 100%, which is extremely accurate). If the conviction of their belief is less than 100%, the user can then be asked to explore the reasons why they think their belief is accurate and also why they believe it might not be. The belief can then be reformulated as being an understandable response to a particular experience. If the user is certain that their belief is true, it may be advisable not to go into this in detail but to spend time exploring alternative potential coping strategies.

Looking forward (maintenance of change)

In order to help users develop an understanding of the long-term need for medication, they can be invited to set themselves a goal or target that they would like to achieve, identify any potential barriers that might get in the way that need to be addressed and how medication might help to achieve their ends. A problem-solving approach can then be used to identify broad and specific tasks that need to be undertaken. This approach affords the opportunity to talk about the importance of maintenance treatment. It also helps to build the user's confidence that they will be able to achieve those outcomes and shows that medication can be part of an enabling process to achieve a goal rather than a disabling process that some patients see medication as being. It is also useful at this point to discuss with the service user their choice of treatment should relapse occur in the future. Users should be given appropriate information about the choices open to them in a realistic and transparent manner.

A medication management case study

The following case study aims to show the use of a medication management approach in a forensic setting and draw the various themes discussed together.

The patient is a 25-year-old single man with a 6-year history of psychotic illness and a coexisting substance use. His offending behaviour included violence towards his parents and members of the public. He was living in a hostel and saw his psychiatrist and care manager regularly.

Engagement

Even though the same multidisciplinary team has been involved in his care for the past 2 years, they found it difficult to engage him in discussing his medication and his intermittent non-adherence. In order to reduce his resistance to talking about medication, the team decided to back off talking about medication for a while and focus more on other aspects of his care for a period of time, such as helping him to sort out his benefits and housing problems. After a number of positive meetings, the subject of taking medication was gradually introduced. Structure was then introduced to the meetings and a collaborative agenda was agreed at the beginning of each session. It was suggested that it would be useful for the team to gain a better understanding of the patient's current views of his medication and his experiences of treatment over the past 6 years.

Summary of assessment

The patient was prescribed a newer antipsychotic to be taken by mouth once a day at night. He saw his psychiatrist every 4 weeks when a new prescription was due. A local chemist supplied his medication but he often forgot or chose not to collect the prescription, resulting in him taking his medication erratically. As a result, his symptoms were not well controlled and he became very distressed by the voices he heard. In the past, his voices have told him to harm people. He admitted to drinking 2–6 cans of beer a day as he believed that this helped him to cope with the voices. He also smoked four joints of cannabis a day and said that this helped him to feel relaxed. The patient had been on his current prescription for 2 years but was unhappy about the weight he had put on since he started taking it. He also described feeling tired a lot of the time. He did not believe he had a mental illness and expressed the view that the doctors had prescribed medication to control him. He also believed that he did not need to take medication when he was not experiencing symptoms.

Medication management interventions

The patient was invited to spend time looking back over his treatment experiences. He was given the opportunity to talk about the negative side of these at length and was told that he could begin his story at any point he wished. He chose to commence from when he was 16 and had started drinking alcohol to cope with longstanding difficulties at home. He described starting smoking cannabis a year later and developing his first episode of mental illness whilst on holiday with his friends. He had tried to jump off a bridge in response to the belief that his friends had turned against him and wanted to kill him.

He had seen a psychiatrist on his return home and was prescribed medication to be taken twice a day. He accepted this for a couple of months but stopped taking it when he felt less scared of people, and also because it made him feel stiff and his hands shook. He still experienced feelings of paranoia and used alcohol to cope with these. He managed to complete the first term of a course at college but had to stop when he punched one of his classmates who he believed could read his thoughts and was interfering with them. This led to his first admission to hospital that lasted 3 months. He described this as a terrifying experience as he was taken there by the police and restrained and injected. He remembered feeling scared of other patients and staff, and had his first experience of hearing disembodied voices during this admission. He was discharged on depot medication that he remained on for 3 years. During this period, he frequently failed to turn up at the mental health centre for his injections or would not answer the door when his nurse called. He was also drinking heavily and smoking cannabis. He frequently got into fights with people in response to his beliefs that they were saying abusive things about him. His voices told him that his family wanted to harm him, also resulting in violence. He was detained under the Mental Health Act and had three admissions to locked psychiatric units. When, during one of these, his medication was changed initially he had a positive view of the new medicine as it helped reduce his voices, made him feel less suspicious of people and he felt more in control of his life. He returned to college to resume his studies but also stopped taking the antipsychotic, as he felt well and believed his symptoms would not return. Unfortunately, they did, which resulted in him seriously assaulting a close relative. At that point, he had his first involvement with forensic services. Assertive follow-up kept him engaged with services but he continued to take his oral medication erratically because of his ongoing concerns about its side effects and his belief that he did not need to take it when well.

Exploring ambivalence

It was explained to the patient that it is normal to be uncertain about taking medication and that people have their own unique reasons for this. He was asked if he wanted to spend some time talking about the not so good things about taking his medication and the good things. The not so good things included feeling hungry, putting on weight and being tired. It was difficult for him to think of anything good initially, but when some of the less obvious benefits were explored he was able to acknowledge that when he did take medication he was less distressed by his voices.

This man's use of alcohol and cannabis were also considered, and the good things and not so good things about them were discussed.

Beliefs about medication

The patient did not believe he needed to take medication once he felt better. He was 70% certain that this was the case. He believed that, when the experiences of the voices and the thinking that people wanted to harm him stopped for a few days, he had conquered them and they would never return. He also thought that alcohol and cannabis were good for relieving stress. He agreed to monitor his voices over the course of a week and rate how distressed he was by them. He was also asked to record each time he took his medication, drank alcohol or smoked cannabis. The following week, he was asked if he would try and take his medication as it is prescribed for the whole week, even if he did not have any symptoms, and monitor the effect on his voices. In the first week, he only took his medication for 2 days and was distressed by what the voices were saying. In the second week, he managed to take his medication every day. After 3 days, he stopped hearing the voices but continued to take the medication, and also recorded that he drank less alcohol. He re-rated his belief that he did not need to take medication once he felt better. This went from having been 70% to only 40% certain that he did not need prescribed medication.

Looking forward

The patient wanted to return to college and finish his studies. He was able to see that he had been successful in staying in college in the past with appropriate support. He also identified that, when he had stopped taking medication, he had become more suspicious of his classmates and got into fights. Learning from the past enabled him to set up a support system to help him get back to his studies. This included being more organised about collecting his medication from the chemist. He also allowed people to remind him that, if he took it continuously it would help him to stay well, and that, if he worked together with the team, his concerns about side effects could be addressed.

CONCLUSION AND KEY POINTS FOR PRACTICE

Aiming to place users and carers at the centre of treatment planning and medication management within a forensic setting is a task for the whole multidisciplinary team. Good medication management practice is based on collaboration, a comprehensive assessment, user-focused problem- and goal-related statements, motivational interviewing and cognitive behavioural interventions, which can produce improved outcomes for service users and their carers.

Medication management is a technique, which can help in assisting service users and others who may be involved to appreciate the need for this form of treatment by working in a collaborative manner with clinical team members. It is an approach that can and should be very much a part of multidisciplinary team working. It may be a very important means of engaging with forensic patients in a potentially very difficult area, particularly in the longer term, but also with very clear benefits, both directly for the individual concerned, and also for those around them and the wider community.

References

Barkley C (2000) Treatment resistance. In Mercer D, Mason T, McKeown M and McCann G (eds) Forensic mental health care: a case study approach. Edinburgh: Churchill Livingstone

Barnes T R E (1989) A rating scale for drug induced akathisia. British Journal of Psychiatry 154: 672–676

Birchwood M, Smith J, Drury V, Healy J, Macmillan F and Slade M (1994) A self-report insight scale for psychosis: reliability, validity and sensitivity to change. Acta Psychiatrica Scandinavica 89: 62–67

Day J C, Wood G, Dewey M and Bentall R P (1995) A self-rating scale for measuring neuroleptic side-effects. Validation in a group of schizophrenic patients. British Journal of Psychiatry 166: 650–653

Department of Health (1999) The National Service framework for mental health. London: The Stationary Office

Gray R (2000) Does patient education enhance compliance with clozapine? A preliminary investigation. Journal of Psychiatric and Mental Health Nursing 7: 285–286

Gray R (2001a) Medication for schizophrenia. Nursing Times 97: 38–39

Gray (2001b) Medication-related cardiac risks and sudden deaths among people receiving antipsychotics for schizophrenia. Mental Health Care 4: 302–304

Gray R, Wykes T and Gournay K (2002) From compliance to concordance: a review of the literature on interventions to enhance compliance with anti-psychotic medication. Journal of Psychiatric and Mental Health Nursing 9: 277–284

Guy W (1976) Assessment manual for psychopharmacology. Washington, DC: Department of Education and Welfare

Hogan T P, Awad A G and Eastwood R (1983) A self-report scale predictive of drug compliance in schizophrenic: reliability and discriminative validity. Psychological Medicine 13: 177–183

Kemp R, Kirov G, Everitt B, Haywood P and David A (1998) Randomised controlled trial for compliance therapy: 18 month follow up. British Journal of Psychiatry 172: 413–419

Lancashire S (1998) KGVM Symptom Scale. Version 6.2. London: Institute of Psychiatry, Kings College London

Lingiarde O, Ahlfors U G, Beck P, Dencker S J and Elsen K (1987) The UKU side effect rating scale. A new comprehensive scale for psychotropic drugs and a cross sectional study of the side effects in neuroleptic treated patients. Acta Psychiatrica Scandinavica (Suppl) 334: 1–100

Macpherson R, Jerrom B and Hughes A (1996) A controlled study of education and drug treatment in schizophrenia. British Journal of Psychiatry 168: 709–717

Marder S R (1999) Anti-psychotic drugs and relapse prevention. Schizophrenia Research 35: Suppl S87–S92

NICE (2002) Guidance on the use of newer (atypical) anti-psychotic drugs for the treatment of schizophrenia. London: National Institute for Clinical Excellence

NICE (2003) Core interventions in the treatment and management of schizophrenia in primary and secondary care. London: National Institute for Clinical Excellence

Pilowsky L S, Costa D C, Ell P J (1992) Clozapine, single photon emission tomography and the D2 dopamine receptor blockade hypothesis of schizophrenia. Lancet 340: 199–202

Taylor D, Paton C and Kerwin R (2003) The South London and Maudsley NHS Trust prescribing guidelines, 7th edn. London: Martin Dunitz

Wieden P and Olfson M (1995) Cost of relapse in schizophrenia. Schizophrenia Bulletin 21: 419–429

Further reading

Haynes P, Montagne P, Oliver T, et al. (2002) Interventions for helping users follow prescriptions for medications (Cochrane Review). In: Cochrane library, Issue 4. Oxford: Update Software

Kemp R, Kirov GD, et al. (1998) Randomised controlled trial of compliance therapy. 18 month follow-up Evertt, British Journal of Psychiatry 172: 413–419

Miller W R (1995) What is motivational interviewing? Behavioural and Cognitive Psychotherapy 23: 325–334

Ohlsen R, Smith S, Taylor D and Pilowsky L (2003) The Maudsley anti-psychotic medication review: service guidelines. London: Martin Dunitz

Taylor D, Paton C and Kerwin R (2003) The South London and Maudsley NHS Trust prescribing guidelines, 7th edn. London: Martin Dunitz

Chapter **10**

Team building

Stuart Wix

CHAPTER CONTENTS

INTRODUCTION

We spent hours in teambuilding exercises - playing tambourines and beating drums together, all making fools of ourselves and joining in to break down barriers . . .

. . . Rugby is a team game and whatever I have achieved, it has been down to fourteen other guys as much as me

Martin Johnson (2003)

These are the prophetic prose of a visionary England rugby captain, who demonstrated the importance of teamwork and a recognition of the differing strengths of his 'team mates', who ultimately succeeded by winning the Rugby World Cup in Australia in 2003. The importance of effective teamwork applies to many sections of our society, where the best and most desirable outcome is sought.

For effective multidisciplinary working within a forensic mental health care system, it is vital to ensure that each individual patient receives the most efficacious care and treatment whilst maintaining a level of security that ensures the safety of all the disciplines involved. At the heart of effective multidisciplinary collaboration lies the implicit expectation that the very safety of the patient and staff group, as well as visitors and the wider public, may well depend on a consistent and shared agreement about how to tackle the risks and issues relating to particular individuals (Burrow, 1999).

However, it is clear that effective team working does not come about by accident or by mere coincidence, as in the case of the 2003 World Cup-winning England rugby team. Yet the majority of professionals engaged in providing effective health care, whose goal is to provide positive health outcomes for patients, recognise the worth of team building in order to enhance collaboration and team functioning (West, 1994; Gorman, 1998; Burrow, 1999; Kirby and Myers, 2000). This chapter will examine how multidisciplinary teams can enhance team functioning through team-building activities by exploring a range of models and team exercises that promote greater cohesiveness. In addition, a range of teamwork-based measuring instruments will be outlined, which may be variously used to provide the team with feedback, and also assist with team development over time.

BUILDING AN EFFECTIVE TEAM

According to West (1994), most team-building interventions are founded upon team relationships and cohesiveness, with the mistaken assumption that enhancements in cohesiveness lead to improvements in team task performance. He further asserts that a few days spent away team building does not necessarily lead to a dramatic improvement in team functioning, in the same way that one session of psychotherapy on its own does not change a person's life. Rather, evidence suggests that regular interaction and effort, through structured and semistructured team building 'away days' is more likely to lead to improvements in functioning.

Away days

The principle of 'away days' for the purposes of team building is a well-established activity within the NHS and other public sector services, as well as private organisations. However, there is a paucity of literature, which adequately, and accurately, describes this activity. The following principles should be observed when teams are considering arranging an 'away day' for the purpose of team building.

- Away days should be held at a venue away from the clinical area.
- The venue should be as informal as possible, to help team members feel relaxed and comfortable.
- Team members' diaries should be clear of all other commitments, with the away day taking precedence.
- All team members should attend.
- All team members must be committed to the day and have appropriate cover for other work.
- The agenda for the away day can be either informal or formal, and agreed in advance by all members of the team.
- The recording of minutes or notes should also be agreed in advance and, if used, should subsequently be circulated to all team members.
- It is also important for there to be a social aspect to the day. It is preferable to schedule the 'social' element of the away day following completion of the team task(s), to promote informality, and encourage more cordial team relationships.

Guidelines for increasing group effectiveness

West (1994) offers a range of guidelines that can lead to an increase in group or team effectiveness:

- groups should have intrinsically interesting tasks to perform;
- individuals should feel they are important to the fate of the group;
- individuals should have intrinsically interesting tasks to perform;
- individual contributions should be indispensable, unique and evaluated against a standard;
- there should be clear team goals with built-in performance feedback.

Groups should have intrinsically interesting tasks to perform

Teams that have an inherently interesting task to perform often generate high commitment, higher motivation and more collaboration from their members. Individuals will work harder if the tasks they are to perform are intrinsically of interest, are motivating, challenging and enjoyable. Teams should, therefore, work on identifying tasks that fit this profile but should also be given considerable autonomy in modifying task objectives to ensure that the team's goals help to maintain overall motivation.

Individuals should feel they are important to the fate of the group

An example of how individuals can come to feel that their work is important to the fate of the group is through the use of techniques of role clarification and negotiation. By careful exploration of the roles of each team member, together with the identification of team and individual objectives, team members can see and demonstrate more clearly to other team members the importance of their own work to the success of the team overall.

Individuals should have intrinsically interesting tasks to perform

Tasks undertaken by each individual member of the team should be meaningful and inherently rewarding. Individual team members will work harder and be more committed and creative, if the tasks they are performing are both challenging and engaging.

Individual contributions should be indispensable, unique and evaluated against a standard

It is extremely important that individual team members' work should be subject to evaluation. Individuals need to feel that their contribution is valued, but also that their performance is visible to other members of the team. For a multidisciplinary team working within a forensic setting, the team members' performance may be measured by such things as the number of inpatients or outpatients seen, the number of assessments undertaken, the average inpatient length of stay, patient satisfaction and patient complaints, the quality of clinical interactions with patients, and the quantity and quality of communications with other team members.

There should be clear team goals with built-in performance feedback

Where individual team members are set clear targets, their performance is likely in general to be improved. However, clear team goals can only function as a motivator of team performance if accurate performance feedback is available. For forensic multidisciplinary teams, there should be performance feedback at least annually on all or some of the following indices:

- patients' satisfaction with the quality of care given;
- effectiveness of innovations and changes introduced by the team;
- quality of care given in the team;
- improvement in mental health of patients;
- the effectiveness with which they have achieved their own objectives as a team;
- quality of intrateam communications;
- quality of relationships with other agencies, such as the probation services and prisons, the Home Office and other referral agencies within the team's catchment area;
- improvement in patient care pathways from higher to the least restrictive environment possible;
- improvement in patient access to physical health care and health promotion in general.

The more precise the indicators of a team's performance are, the more likely it is to improve its performance (West, 1994).

MEASUREMENT OF TEAM PERFORMANCE

An audit tool developed by Borrill and West (2001) is designed to help teams working in the NHS function together more effectively. It is intended to allow teams to assess how well they are working together. The measure includes a number of statements that could describe a team (Table 10.1). A group is asked to indicate how accurately they think each statement describes the team in which they currently work most of the time.

Borrill and West (2001) suggest that team members calculate their individual score for each subset of questions by writing the rating (1, 2, 3, 4 or 5) for each question on the scoring sheet. These are then added together to display the total score for each cumulative area, such as decision-making and communication (questions 4, 6, 7, 8 and 16). For each subset, the total score is then divided by the number of questions to calculate the average figure. For example, to calculate the mean score for the area 'Clarity of commitment to team objectives', the ratings are added together for questions 1, 10 and 12, and then divided by the number of questions, namely three (see Table 10.2).

Total scores can then be calculated for the team as a whole for each area. To do this, the average scores are totalled for each area from every individual team member. The average score is then calculated for the team on each area by dividing the total for the team by the number of team members who completed the questionnaire (Table 10.3).

TEAM PERFORMANCE AND PERSONALITY TYPE

In order for a multidisciplinary team to function and for its members to interact effectively, it can sometimes prove invaluable for them to obtain an understanding of one another's differences during 'start up' sessions, preferably when a team comes together for the first time. One of the most respected psychometric instruments and possibly one of the oldest is the

Table 10.1 Team working questionnaire

	Very inaccurate description 1	Inaccurate description 2	Somewhat accurate 3	Accurate description 4	Very accurate description 5
1. In this team we are clear about what we are trying to achieve					
2. We know we can rely on one another in this team					
3. We have lively debates about how best to do the work					
4. We meet together sufficiently frequently to ensure effective communication and cooperation					
5. People in the team are quick to offer help to try out new ways of doing things					
6. We all influence the final decisions made in the team					
7. We are careful to keep each other informed about work issues					
8. There is a feeling of trust and safety in this team					
9. We are enthusiastic about innovation in this team					
10. Team members are committed to achieving the team's objectives					
11. We can safely discuss errors and mistakes in the team					
12. We agree in the team about what are our team objectives					
13. There is a climate of constructive criticism in this team					
14. We support each other in ideas for new and improved ways of doing the team's work					
15. We work supportively together to get the job done					
16. Everyone in the team contributes to decision-making					

Myers–Briggs type indicator (MBTI), which is used extensively around the world. The indicator is designed to make Carl Jung's theory of psychological types understandable and useful when considering team-building activity. Its benefit is in providing a quick method in helping teams understand themselves as individuals and other team members better by getting to their thinking preferences. In short, the MBTI inventory will assist individuals with their motivations, natural strengths and potential areas for growth, whilst at the same time helping them to appreciate other team members who differ from them, thus encouraging cooperation with others and reducing the potential for miscommunication (Kirby and Myers, 2000).

Table 10.2 Individual team scoring sheet

	Question		Question
Clarity and commitment to team objectives	1 10 12 Total Average (Total divided by 3)	Focus on quality	3 11 13 15 Total Average (Total divided by 4)
Decision-making and communication	4 6 7 8 16 Total Average (Total divided by 5)	Support for innovation	2 5 9 14 Total Average (Total divided by 4)

Table 10.3 Team scoring sheet

	Total for team	Team average
Clarity and commitment to team objectives		
Decision-making and communication		
Focus on quality		
Support for innovation		
Total scores		

According to Kirby and Myers (2000), there are eight fundamental thinking preferences that can be located in the MBTI, which are organised into four bipolar scales (see Table 10.4).

Use of the MBTI personality inventory by teams has grown rapidly in the last decade, as leaders and employees have come to recognise its practical usefulness in solving team problems. Kirby and Myers (2000) argue that psychological type as identified by the MBTI provides the following benefits for teams.

1. MBTI results and interpretation focus on how people take in information (perception) and how they prioritise that information to make decisions (judgement)—basic personality facets that underlie most tasks and training.
2. MBTI type enhances people's clarity about and comfort with their own work styles, while constructively identifying possible blind spots and areas of vulnerability.
3. Type theory and the MBTI give a logical coherent structure for understanding normal differences between people in a host of different areas, including working in teams.

Table 10.4   The four scales (MBTI) (Kirby and Myers, 2000)

Energising	Extraversion (E)	Introversion (I)
Unconscious preoccupation	Drawing energy from the world of people, things, activities, dealing in breadth rather than depth Access to people	Drawing energy from the internal world of thoughts, ideas, preferring depth; pausing for thought Privacy
Perceiving	**Sensing (S)**	**Intuition (N)**
Unconscious preoccupation	Preferring to take in information through the five senses, liking the concrete and practical; tolerating detail Evidence	Preferring to take in information through a sixth sense of what might be; like the big picture; tolerating change Possibilities
Decision–making	**Thinking (T)**	**Feeling (F)**
Unconscious preoccupation	Structuring decisions through objective tolerance, emphasising logic and reason, truth and fairness Truth	Structuring decisions through an emphasis on personal values, people's needs Harmony with others
Living	**Judging (J)**	**Perceiving (P)**
Unconscious preoccupation	Preferring to live in a planned, organised way; liking to come to conclusions quickly Control	Preferring to live in a spontaneous, flexible way, adapting rather than controlling Keeping options open

4. Type theory presents a dynamic picture of individual functioning, including recognition of the dominant function as the basis of motivating and identification of customary responses to stress.
5. Type theory outlines a model of lifelong individual development, and the MBTI identifies likely paths for development useful with teams and in coaching individual leaders.
6. The MBTI provides a perspective and data for analysing organisational culture, management structures and other organisational systems.
7. The MBTI and supporting type resources demonstrate the value added by diversity within the organization or team. This ethic—the constructive use of differences—is particularly applicable in today's global and diverse forms of team working.

When conducting a Myers–Briggs workshop whilst team building, it is preferable to enlist the assistance of a suitably trained individual, who may be any competent professional from within the organisation. The MBTI is not a tool that can be simply picked up and used immediately by the uninitiated, yet it can be extremely informative, if an experienced practitioner who has the knowledge necessary for accurate and appropriate interpretation facilitates its use.

TEAM–BUILDING INTERVENTIONS

According to West (1994), team-building interventions can be divided into five main types, each requiring a particular approach:

1. team start-up;
2. regular formal reviews;
3. addressing known task-related problems;
4. identifying what the problems are;
5. social process interventions.

1. Team start-up

West asserts that the beginning of a team's life has a significant influence on its later development and effectiveness, especially when a crisis occurs. Effort should go into determining the overall task and objectives for the team, clarifying objectives and inter-related roles for team members and the team as a whole, and establishing mechanisms for regular communication and review of all aspects of team functioning (West, 1994).

The British Psychological Society (1991) suggests that teams should employ a checklist of questions during 'start-up' to help clarify individual roles and team objectives. For instance:

- Are all team members clear about the purpose of the team?
- Has the amount of time to be spent on team objectives by team members been agreed?
- Who are the target clients for the team?
- Is the team's role to provide a direct client service or indirect services (such as education, training, etc.) or both?
- Have service priorities been agreed?
- Have issues of leadership been resolved?
- How are the team members to be coordinated? For example, by an administrative coordinator, or on the basis of members taking prime responsibility according to the needs of the case or by a team leader?
- Who sets the limits for individual workloads?
- Who monitors or collates the work of the team as a whole?
- Has a policy been agreed for referrals to the team and allocation of work within the team?
- Has a procedure been agreed for care planning and case review?
- Has a procedure been agreed for discontinuing individual participation in a case and discharge from team involvement?
- Has a procedure been agreed for transfer of a case from one member to another?
- Have the skills and responsibilities of team members been identified?
- Are team members clear about what they are accountable for and to whom?
- Have 'dual influences' (i.e. responsibilities to team and line managers) been clarified for each profession?
- Who decides on withdrawal or replacements of team members?
- Has a procedure been agreed for obtaining clients' or guardians' consent to the sharing of confidential information within the team?
- Has a policy been agreed on passing information to people outside the team, especially, for instance, across agencies?

2. Regular formal reviews

According to West (1994), all team members should attend away days, which must be carefully planned with a sufficient degree of flexibility to allow emerging topics to be dealt with appropriately. He also argues that, where possible, a team should consider the commissioning of a facilitator to enable team leaders and other team members to focus on the content of the day. Topics to be covered on away days might include the following:

- team successes and difficulties in the previous 6-month or 1-year period;
- a review of team objectives and their appropriateness;
- the roles of team members;
- quality of team communication;
- team interaction frequency;
- team decision-making processes;
- excellence in the team's work;
- support for innovation;
- team social support;
- conflict resolution in the team;
- support for personal growth and development.

3. Addressing known task-related problems

West argues that, where a specific problem can be identified that team members have identified correctly, it is useful for the team to take time out for focused intervention. The most desirable outcome can be best achieved with the assistance of a facilitator, who can help the team develop alternative options for overcoming the problem and action plans for implementing the selected way forward.

4. Identifying what the problems are

Following on from addressing known task-related problems, West suggests that the intervention focuses on the team identifying appropriate strategies to overcome specific problems. This can be achieved in a range of ways from extended group discussion to employing a questionnaire measure that can be used as a diagnostic instrument to identify problems in team functioning and as an aid to identifying techniques associated with particular team problems.

5. Social process interventions

West recommends that team social process interventions should be employed where a team has unsatisfactory answers to one or more of the questions listed in Table 10.5. Interventions should focus on one area rather than attempting to accomplish change in all. For example, if a problem relates to a failure to resolve conflicts in a timely fashion, a conflict resolution technique based on the principles of assertiveness and ethical negotiation can be introduced.

ROLE CLARIFICATION AND NEGOTIATION

West asserts that a potential difficulty for teams is sometimes the lack of clarity regarding team roles. Team members may fear that such questioning may generate conflict about the team's direction. However, research evidence regarding reflexivity suggests the reverse, where teams who

Table 10.5 West's satisfaction with team social processes

	Yes, very definitely	Yes, but only somewhat	No, but only somewhat	No, definitely not
Does the team provide adequate levels of social support for its members?	1	2	3	4
Does the team have constructive, healthy approaches to conflict resolution?	1	2	3	4
Does the team have a generally warm and positive social climate?	1	2	3	4
Does the team provide adequate support for skill development, training and personal development of all its members?	1	2	3	4

Have the whole team discuss team scores on this questionnaire and discuss whether there is a need to improve any of those areas of team social functioning

manage to reflect on strategies in this way are more effective in terms of long-term performance. West recommends a role negotiation exercise for teams to assist team members with this process (see Table 10.6).

For those teams that might consider West's approach to team building too rigid and prescriptive, they may find a rather more eclectic view, such as that described by Gorman (1998), more acceptable. In his book, *'Managing multi-disciplinary teams in the NHS'*, Gorman suggests that team building can only commence once team members have a greater understanding of team dynamics, which is illustrated with the basic life cycle of a team, where he cites Tuckman's formula of the 1960s (Tuckman, 1965). Tuckman argues that most teams tend to have four phases in their life cycle (see Figure 10.1).

Figure 10.1 Tuckman's life cycle of a team

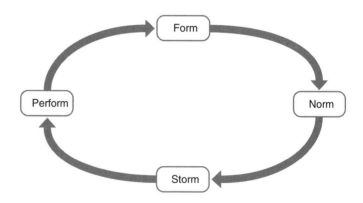

THE BASIC LIFE CYCLE OF A TEAM

Tuckman's formula begins with the first phase 'form', which involves getting to know each other, where team members begin to explore roles and the task. The next phase is 'norm', that is developing formal or informal rules of conduct and behaviour that will govern the way the team will work together. 'Storm' is the third phase, where conflict begins

Table 10.6 West's role negotiation exercise

Team members use mutual influence and negotiation in order to change team behaviours and improve team functioning

Step 1

Each team member lists his or her objectives and principal activities on a piece of flip chart paper

Step 2

Each piece of flip chart paper is hung on the wall around the room and team members examine each role

Step 3

Under three headings on a piece of paper, each team member writes down what behaviours they would like that person to do less, do more, or maintain at the present level in their working relationship. For example, a receptionist might indicate that they want a particular GP to keep them informed more fully of plans for the coming month, in order that they are not inappropriately ignorant of the GP's movements. The receptionist may ask the GP not to check so often the patients' paperwork has been completed, since it feels like controlling rather than trusting their role. Finally, he or she may ask the GP to sustain these attempts to involve the receptionist in decisions concerning the general running of the practice.
Each person signs their name after their requests for more, less or maintained behaviour

Step 4

Pairs of individuals within the team then meet to examine the end result. The two negotiate together in order to reach agreement about the various requests. This is a highly participate step in the exercise and some teams may need help in managing the negotiation, especially if a particular pair is having difficulty reaching agreement. Through role negotiation, the needs of individual roles are met more effectively and the functioning of individual members is dovetailed more into the objective and needs of the team as a whole. This is a very powerful exercise, which can enhance team functioning considerably, overcoming many of the problems of process loss and coordination

between individuals about roles, priorities and relationships. In the final phase, 'perform', it is postulated, having finally 'cleared the air', the team is able to 'perform', and also carry out tasks efficiently and effectively (Gorman, 1998).

GORMAN'S APPROACHES

Gorman also outlines six different approaches that multidisciplinary teams may utilise as part of a process of team building and learning. These are described as:

- action learning;
- clinical audit;
- PUNS and STUNS;
- shadowing;

- peer review;
- 360-degree feedback.

Action learning

Gorman asserts that action learning can be particularly useful, as it focuses upon the development of questioning knowledge through discussion with peers and colleagues. Action learning often takes place in small groups, sometimes called action learning sets, which meet regularly over a period of time, whose purpose is to work on real problems and issues brought by its members. He suggests that action learning can be a powerful technique, as it is very closely allied to action research, and is based on the type of discussions that practitioners will have with their peers about specific problems and issues. Action learning, therefore, has a focus on these discussions, ensuring that they occur in a structured and supported way.

The objective of action learning is to encourage team members to reflect critically on their practice, to challenge each other by giving and receiving feedback, and to work through feelings about individual, sometimes complex and paradoxical roles. A typical action learning process might be the following.

- *Individual check-in* (2–3 minutes from each team member, summarising what has happened since the last team meeting—total 20 minutes).
- *Check-in* with individuals who 'worked' at the last meeting to offer brief reports on the progress of the issue since the last away day and the learning to be gained from that (20 minutes).
- *Bid for space*, determining which team member wishes to work on this occasion (10 minutes).
- *Process time*—three sessions of 45 minutes with break of 10 minutes (145 minutes).
- *Review of team process,* and ending of team meeting (up to 15 minutes).

To summarise, action learning promotes the following.

- It values everyone.
- It is democratic.
- It stresses questions.
- It insists on actions.
- It gives courage.
- It encourages responsibility.
- It examines everything.

Clinical audit

Clinical audit, which is a key component of clinical governance, focuses upon measuring the effectiveness of clinical procedures (Gorman, 1998). Audit techniques usually start with a defined standard or norm of performance, where the actual performance is then compared to this defined standard. Deficiencies are identified and action by the team is taken to remedy them. Clinical audit can help to bring about debates within a multidisciplinary team about service priority and how tangible improvement can be brought about in relation to patient care.

PUNS and STUNS

According to Gorman, PUNS (patient unmet needs) and STUNS (staff unmet needs) can be utilised as a critical incident analysis approach to identifying patient and staff unmet need, which he originally developed for use in general practice. He described the process, which works by asking staff in a meeting to give examples they have observed where a patient has had an unmet need as a result of the way the service was organised, or because of the knowledge or lack of knowledge of staff. The underlying causes are then discussed and actions agreed to remedy them. Gorman argues that the process of PUNS and STUNS is a good way of validating staff knowledge and as a mechanism also of observing patterns that may emerge over time. He suggests that this technique can have positive as well as negative effects on a multidisciplinary team. Its advantage lies in the fact that practice is explored with a colleague who shares expertise and inclination. The potential disadvantage of this technique for teams lies, of course, in the fact that it can reinforce the unidisciplinary nature of most professional training and education for each of the individual team members (Gorman, 1998).

Shadowing

According to Gorman, shadowing, accompanying a fellow team member in their day-to-day work, is a technique that is useful in the early stages of a multidisciplinary teams' development, particularly where one team member is trying to understand the specific role of a colleague and the constraints under which they may be operating. However, a potential weakness of this form of exercise is that it may be time consuming and heavy on human and, therefore, clinical resources.

360–degree feedback

The final approach described by Gorman, as part of the team-building process, is that of 360-degree feedback, something that has already attained greater prominence in the NHS in recent years as a part of professional appraisal and commentary on performance. He describes 360-degree feedback as a process by which individuals attain feedback from their managers, peers in the team and others with whom they are in contact, including, of course, patients or service users and consumers, as well as carers and relatives. In short, the feedback comes from all directions, above, below and sideways. Gorman (1998) asserts that this technique can provide powerful insights into how a multidisciplinary team is operating as a whole, by revisiting questions such as 'Have professional boundaries been broken down?' or 'Are team members clear about their role and purpose?' and 'Do they feel part of a team?'

As teams strive to develop and improve collaboration and effective multidisciplinary working, the need for focused, informative and helpful feedback becomes essential. Integrating them with the team's personal and professional development planning, and making them an annual event frequently sustain feedback, utilising a 360-degree approach. The benefits of 360-degree feedback can be summarised as shown in Table 10.7.

Table 10.7 The benefits of 360-degree feedback

For the individual

Promotes the development of more considered, focused and effective personal development plans
Feedback from all directions gives a truly rounded view of performance
Confidential process promotes more honest feedback
Provides benchmarks against performance of a team
Can reinvigorate stalled careers

For the team

Framework aligns the feedback to the purpose objectives and values of the team
Promotes a performance culture within the team
A powerful tool, which can be used as part of an organised change process
Signals a real and substantial interest in the development of individuals

It is very important, when implementing 360-degree feedback with a multidisciplinary team, to be sensitive, as some individual team members might think of this approach as threatening. To overcome potential concerns, it is sometimes useful to give team members a careful briefing, ensuring that there is no sense in which the system will be used to persecute individuals, encouraging them to be as candid as possible without fear of recrimination.

The strength of Gorman's eclectic approach to team building can be located in his experience and knowledge of the NHS as an organisation, and that most of the examples he gives are based upon previous practical application when working with teams.

CONCLUSION

This chapter has attempted to outline some examples of focused team-building activity, although it is by no means exhaustive. There are other models that exist in the literature (see Bassett and Brunning, 1989; Cordess, 1996).

The importance of team building as a regular activity for forensic multidisciplinary teams cannot be underestimated. The team imperative, as a result of productive team building, is far greater collaborative integrity in targeting offending behaviour in the context of psychiatric morbidity. This collaboration, within a forensic mental health context, brings with it the inevitable demand of security considerations that maintain a safe environment in which a multidisciplinary team operates but also an enhanced sense of shared responsibility and purpose when working in a potentially stressful field.

Through greater shared understanding of one another's role, personality type (Kirby and Myers, 2000) and the use of systematic team-building techniques over time, as described in this chapter, the forensic clinical team can develop and grow to meet the challenging demands of its patient population. Forensic clinical teams, as a function of team building, can, therefore, invest more collaboratively in the process of ongoing assessment, therapeutic intervention, review, expert advice, care pathway planning, and training and education. There is also an implicit expectation that patients and carers themselves are actively involved with this process, in collaborating with a team when planning and evaluating their care.

References

Bassett T and Brunning H (1989) Power stations, a workshop exploring the issue of power in multidisciplinary teams. Brighton: Pavilion Publishing

Borrill C and West M (2001) How good is your team? A guide for team members. London: Department of Health

British Psychological Society (1991) Responsibility issues in clinical psychology and multi-disciplinary teamwork. London: British Psychological Society

Burrow S (1999) The forensic multi-disciplinary care team. In: Tarbuck P, Topping-Morris B and Burnard P (eds) Forensic mental health nursing, strategy and implication. London: Whurr Publishers

Cordess C (1996) The multi-disciplinary team. In: Cordess C and Cox M (eds) Forensic psychotherapy: crime, psychodynamics and the offender patient. London: Jessica Kingsley

Gorman P (1998) Managing multi-disciplinary teams in the NHS. Milton Keynes: Open University Press

Johnson M (2003) Martin Johnson, the autobiography. London: Headline Book Publishing

Kirby L and Myers K (2000) Introduction to type. Oxford: Oxford Psychological Press

Tuckman B (1965) Development sequences in small groups. Psychological Bulletin 63: 384–389

West MA (1994) Effective team work. London: British Psychological Society

Chapter 11

Multidisciplinary training and education

Stuart Wix and Martin Humphreys

INTRODUCTION

Traditionally, education in health care has been considered in terms of individual professional development occurring within separate physical environments or departments. Additionally, continuing professional development (CPD) has been considered as a process that occurs within each discipline or profession, and which is monitored by and within that same professional group. This model of education presents a particular issue for an individual, whose professional framework is not necessarily associated closely with the demands facing the organisation. The National Health Service Executive (NHSE, 1998) in the government circular *Working together* proposed that NHS employers should have in place training and development plans for the majority of professional health service staff. Forensic mental health services, more particularly, are urged to utilise the lessons learned from previous inquiries and incorporate these in plans for local service development. Included within this premise is the identification of failures of care, 'near misses' and consequent public interest and concern. The National Institute for Clinical Excellence (NICE) for instance, has produced a range of guidelines, which will enable forensic mental health professionals to formulate professional development activities. These, in turn, are likely to be integrated within the process of audit of a more sophisticated and far-reaching nature, which, in turn, will be closely linked to national standards and clinical guidelines.

It is the government's aim that employers should align their existing training budgets with service objectives and clinical governance plans, with a clear strategy that enhances learning that is work based. One of the problems in the past has been concern about potentially diluting the individual training of each of the professions and the need for them to maintain their own professional standards, examinations and institutions. Specific requirements of training at undergraduate and postgraduate level may compromise or potentially prevent, multidisciplinary learning until much later in a career, by which time other aspects of work have changed and the opportunity is no longer available or wanted.

The United Kingdom Central Council for Nursing, Midwifery and Health Visiting (UKCC, 1999) has published a document entitled *Nursing in secure environments*, which was produced and researched in partnership with the University of Central Lancashire. In many respects, this publication represented a watershed for forensic mental health nurses across the secure-care spectrum, particularly in regard to post registration education and CPD. Educationalists as well as practitioners, who were considered key informants in organisations, were asked for both qualitative and quantitative information about their preparation, induction and ongoing professional development for working in secure settings. The main issues that emerged from the study related to the following identified deficits:

- clinical supervision;
- induction;
- physical intervention—control and restraint (C and R) training.

Overall, this document highlighted the lack of consistency and strategic development of training and education programmes for nurses within secure settings. Although the focus of the study was mainly around the needs of this particular professional group, there was also an underlying recognition of the organisational deficits, which affected other health care workers within forensic services.

It is vital, therefore, that the various professions link their training and professional development to the expectations of the organisation for which they work. There is a need to identify core competencies and common themes relevant to all practitioners, which include the following (Hope, 1999).

- Developing a more holistic view of the person with mental health problems, and exploring values necessary for building and sustaining effective relationships with users, carers and mental health workers.
- 'Getting the fundamentals right'.
- Giving staff more confidence in areas such as risk assessment and management, crisis intervention, managing confrontation and de-escalation techniques.
- Facilitating training to enable staff to deliver effective interventions and avoid overprotection of clients.
- Facilitating personal and professional development by encouraging reflective practice and the use of clinical supervision.

Clinical governance as a framework for improving quality and standards of clinical care, also strongly reinforces the principle that lifelong learning should be designed to meet the needs of an organisation, as well as the aspirations of contributing professionals (Thompson et al., 2001). Thompson et al. (2001) also suggest that forensic mental health services depend upon the professional workforce to make the organisation function effectively. Furthermore, CPD is considered absolutely vital to support the delivery of high standards of patient care, which are considered key to the medium- to long-term success of a training and education programme for an organisation:

- Development should be participative and the focus should be, or should involve, the practitioner.
- It should be targeted toward direct patient care.
- It should be aimed at meeting an identified educational need.
- It should be based on accurate evidence, which is educationally effective.
- It should be lodged within the wider organisational strategic and development plans.
- It should transfer across the professional and service delivery boundaries.
- It should reflect previous knowledge and experience of practice (Thompson et al., 2001: 74).

A training and education programme within a forensic mental health setting, which has a multidisciplinary emphasis and foundation, can provide a wide range of opportunities as well as advantages for a service. This chapter will outline some of the main themes that influence multiprofessional training and education in forensic mental health services. This will be achieved by examination of a number of scoping studies and key publications, which have provided strategic direction and identified gaps in training provision. In addition, there will be a discussion of the potential for multidisciplinary post-registration higher education programmes for forensic mental health professionals, a consideration of the very topical subject of involving users of services and their carers in teaching and training, and some suggestions for future directions in this field.

TRAINING AND EDUCATION: AN OVERVIEW

Bloom and Parad (1976), in a survey of staff members and training programme directors in Boulder, Colorado, suggest that multidisciplinary functioning is the rule rather than the exception. The study noted a number of advantages of multidisciplinary settings for training community psychologists and indicated that such settings may establish in one place a variety of professional resources for shared problem solving, and went on to state: 'The optimum beneficiaries of multidisciplinary training are persons who have had extensive and diverse professional experience, are emotionally and professionally mature, have a clear personal identity, and really love tackling new and unfamiliar topics and making sense out of them' (Bloom and Parad, 1976: 670).

The authors further suggest that certain types of cooperative activity among the four core mental health disciplines—psychiatry, psychology, mental health nursing and social work—will enhance organisational effectiveness in general and service delivery to patients in particular. According to this view, a small group of mental health staff members of different disciplines, with a shared responsibility, can produce a synergistic effect. That is to say that multidisciplinary team effort can be significantly greater than the cumulative effects of the discrete performance of individual practitioners.

Training by definition implies skills development and/or instruction, which in forensic mental health care and in relation to a number of professional disciplines, require further clarity as to what these skills or competencies might be (Chaloner, 2000). The skills required of professional disciplines have been outlined in the publication entitled *Pulling together* (Sainsbury Centre for Mental Health, 1997), which are summarised as follows.

- There is a clear mismatch between current training arrangements and current and future service needs.
- Core values and competencies need to be established across specialisms and agencies.
- Occupational standards should be developed, linked to core competencies and reflected in training.

From these key points an organisation should develop the following principles:

- the need for a set of core values to underpin all training and development;
- the need for a multidisciplinary approach to the planning and delivery of training;
- the need to consider curricula of current preregistered and postregistered training courses;
- the need to examine the organisational cultures necessary to effect change;
- the need to consider training and support for groups not traditionally covered (e.g. service users and carers, unqualified staff and managers);
- the need for effective mechanisms and networks to share good practices, as although much good practice exists, it is not always comprehensive or widely disseminated.

The Department of Health (1997), in a paper regarding professional development of staff, outlined a range of points to help health organisations achieve the objective of clinical excellence and quality improvement. A keystone of clinical governance to help staff recognise education and training needs, to budget for these needs and to measure outcomes is the requirement of professional development plans as part of the process of appraisal. Thompson et al. (2001) also recognise the strength of a performance management process and assert that it is designed to improve the quality of service delivery. They further suggest that secure services should have the following elements in place:

- an appraisal system;
- monitoring arrangements to identify training and development needs;
- leadership programmes to develop clinical teams;
- a strategy for workforce planning, including lifelong learning.

The production and subsequent utilisation of specific standards that focus upon the CPD needs of professional staff can also serve as a performance management strategy to ensure that these standards are being followed. The 'whole service' approach will help to harmonise practice across the organisation, which serves to identify multidisciplinary training and education gaps and themes, which can help to enhance service delivery over time (see Table 11.1).

TREATMENT INTEGRITY AND ITS RELATIONSHIP TO TRAINING

According to Thomas-Peter (1999) there are two issues frequently associated with the rehabilitation of offenders, firstly that of having to work across boundaries of several agencies in order to provide unified services to a group of individuals with similar needs and, secondly, of managing treatment programmes with a rigour that ensures sufficient quality to maximise the treatment effect, something which has come to be known as a 'treatment integrity'. Both issues are related and can be described as the process by which patients migrate across boundaries of different agencies, or across significant service boundaries in the same agency, where treatment integrity is most likely to be compromised or where the integration of services themselves is poor.

Treatment integrity is where:

- an intervention is derived from what is known to have best results;
- an intervention is clearly specified and has goals;
- an intervention is delivered by staff who have a high level of knowledge;
- the service that is actually delivered is the same as that which is intended to be delivered.

CONDITIONS THAT SUPPORT TREATMENT INTEGRITY

Thomas-Peter (1999) suggests that there are a number of organisational and service conditions that may enhance treatment integrity, which is likely to be improved in the following situations.

1. All agencies and participants agree the purpose of the programme.
2. The priority of addressing this purpose is stated for each agency or operational section, and is acceptable for the other agency or section.
3. The process of developing the programme is agreed and includes all of those, inside and outside of participant agencies, which can affect the success of the intended programme.
4. There is confluence of authority and responsibility for all aspects of the programme within the organisation. In other words, those with the authority or the influence to affect the programme's development

Table 11.1 Continuing professional development standards for a forensic mental health service: staff supervision, appraisal and training

1.1 Supervision/appraisal

1.1.1 Standard: staff have adequate supervision and appraisal

a. Employers ensure that there is a clear supervision and appraisal framework, including adequate defined time, and there is evidence that these functions are carried out regularly, and in accordance with local and professional guidelines

b. There are formal mechanisms, for example, individual supervision and team meetings, in which staff may report to their managers any problems that hinder their effective delivery of care to service users

c. Staff receive regular (i.e. at least monthly) supervision and support, aimed at helping them examine their personal and professional attitudes towards mentally disordered offenders

d. The lead authority ensures that clinical supervisors have sufficient time to engage in planned peer group meetings in which they are given an opportunity to consider and develop strategies for the proper maintenance and delivery of good clinical practice

e. Personal development plans should include an individual's training needs and requirements for each appraisee. Key themes can then be forwarded from each discipline to the CPD subgroup for consideration

1.2 Training

1.2.1 Standard: multidisciplinary training is provided for all staff

a. New staff members receive induction training on the range of health, housing and social services for people with mental health problems, including statutory roles and responsibilities, cultures and protocols

b. Staff receive training in the Mental Health Act 1983, the revised code of practice and other associated legislation and government guidelines

c. Staff are trained in the assessment of risk of harm to others and to self

d. Staff receive training in the management of imminent and actual violence

e. All staff working with mentally disordered offenders have received training in the identification and handling of potentially dangerous or suicidal patients, and of procedures for dealing with violence or threats to staff

f. All clinical staff receive training in breakaway techniques and/or restraint measures as appropriate

g. These staff are offered the opportunity to refresh these skills regularly

h. Key workers have been trained in the core areas of CPA, health and social care needs assessment, matching services and needs, continuing care and involving users

i. Training in CPA is provided for other clinical staff, including secretarial and clerical staff, service managers, purchasers, GPs, voluntary sector, probation, police, users and carers

j. Probation officers who are to act as social supervisors to conditionally discharged forensic patients receive additional, more specialised training

k. Staff working with mentally disordered offenders have received training on understanding the effects of offending, for example, the needs of the victim

l. Staff working with mentally disordered offenders have received training on ethnic minority and gender issues

and performance are also explicitly accountable for its success or failure.

5. There is reference to evidence and theory that guides the development of the programme.

6. The parameters of the programme, such as the expectations, criteria for success and limitations are clearly stated.

7. There are sufficient staff with the necessary expertise to provide the service. Further, those providing the service remain involved at all operational phases of the programme.

8. The programme is insulated from sudden or unpredictable change from outside.
9. There is close supervision of the programme's activities (design, implementation, delivery) and independent professional review.
10. Rehabilitation/treatment services extend beyond institutional care and into the community.

Treatment integrity is, therefore, critically dependent upon the integration of professional training and personal development with organisational needs. The same author (Thomas-Peter, 1999) further suggests that from an organisational perspective, staff might seek to work across agency boundaries where patients are managed by the same staff through the various levels of security and into the community. However, he also recognises the potential difficulties, which may exist with such a Utopian model, which might become evident when attempting to assist the various professions to link their training and professional development with organisational needs, as it is difficult for any service to encompass fully or effectively the traditions of all the disciplines involved in the care and treatment of the mentally disordered offender.

ORGANISING TRAINING PROGRAMMES

Individual professional groups periodically taking a lead on specific areas have largely influenced training within forensic services. Training is also influenced by wider organisational strategies, which have identified priorities for training or have been generated by recommendations that have come out of inquiries following serious incidents and/or directives that relate to government policy. However, training personnel, who often have a professional nursing background, tend predominantly to lead induction programmes. Although a range of disciplines within a forensic service might be involved in such an induction programme, sometimes no clear multidisciplinary strategy exists for this vital activity. A typical range of potential training topic areas for a secure service induction programme, which could be delivered in a multidisciplinary framework might include:

- risk assessment training;
- Mental Health Act (with a specific focus on Part Two of the Act, 1983);
- MAPA (management of actual and potential aggression);
- working with clients who have a personality disorder or, in particular, antisocial or borderline personality disorder;
- CBT training;
- medication/psychopharmacy;
- information technology;
- management of suicide/self-harm;
- research awareness;
- cultural awareness;
- leadership.

A service needs also to have an overview of the mandatory training requirements of all the different professional groups, which might be coordinated by a dedicated multidisciplinary CPD or training and education forum or committee, which can maintain an overview of the service needs and potential gaps, and where individual representations from each professional group can explain the needs and requirements of their own departmental colleagues (see Table 11.2 for an outline example).

The desired outcome of a clear strategic training and education programme for a forensic service will help to create a mental health care delivery system that can meet the needs of patients in a competent style, which is delivered in a more focused manner, that is available at the appropriate time and embedded in a framework of qualifications linked to national occupational standards (Thompson et al., 2001).

MULTIDISCIPLINARY POSTREGISTRATION TRAINING IN FORENSIC MENTAL HEALTH CARE

As an ideal, multidisciplinary postgraduate training in an area such as forensic mental care would be highly desirable, given the nature of the work, and the structures and various functions of multiprofessional teams operating in the field already described. In the United Kingdom, however, there is relatively little in the way of formal opportunities of multidisciplinary training, other than on a local level, at the present time. This is, nevertheless, a developing area and one that might take a variety of different forms. Some of the potential difficulties in envisaging how this type of educational initiative might be taken forward have to do with the varying professional backgrounds of those involved in forensic mental health care, the differences in their undergraduate or pre-registration training programmes, perceptions of roles in multidisciplinary teams, the potential for professional rivalry and problems associated with pitching the delivery of information and its style at a multiprofessional audience. This is all apart from issues to do with the availability of time for busy working professionals, and the financial implications that there might be for the individual concerned or their employer.

There are possibilities for postgraduate training and potential ways in which a multidisciplinary-based course might be set up and run. It is also possible that those working in the forensic mental health field from a variety of different professional backgrounds might wish to take up the opportunity of learning in an allied, but slightly different area, such as the field of criminology or criminal justice studies. Nevertheless, the potential value of multidisciplinary learning in the specific field of forensic mental health care should not be underestimated.

With a relatively flexible approach to entrance requirements and qualifications, which is an inevitable need where one is offering the same course to those with different types of training previously, it is possible to envisage, for instance, masters level postgraduate studies for all of those who might be, or might become part of, a multidisciplinary team in forensic mental health care. This would not involve adjusting or varying the entrance requirements, depending upon the individual's professional group but might, for instance, involve a combination of a professional or degree-level qualification and/or sufficient practical clinical experience previously and current involvement in the field. In this way, there is the opportunity for the inclusion of those from all sorts of areas of work, not necessarily even clinical practitioners alone but those working,

Table 11.2 Overview of mandatory training requirements of different professional groups

Course	Course details and/or information	For whom	Frequency
Forensic two-day induction	Introduction for all new staff to the philosophy of care at Forensic Service. Sessions include: personal safety, breakaway skills, risk assessment, equal opportunities and security	All staff	Essential within 1 month
Department-/unit-based induction	To help the new starter settle into their new working environment and provide them with essential information required for working in a safer manner	All staff	Essential within 6 weeks
Appraisal with personal development plan	For the appraisee to reflect on their achievements over the previous year and in conjunction with their line manager, identify their learning needs for the next 12 months	All staff	Mandatory—yearly
Violence and personal safety: management of actual and potential aggression (MAPA)	To provide the learner with the necessary skills to improve confidence when managing actual or potential aggression	Consultants, AHPs, A&C, facilities staff, estates staff, update for all	1-day course every 2 years
		Medical staff—SHOs, SpRs, staff grades	½-day course annually
		Older adult nurses in RSU and satellite units	3-day course with an annual update
		AHPs, pharmacists, psychologists	3-day course every 2 years
		All frontline nurses and some AHPs	10-day MAPA course with an annual update
MAPA refresher 1-day	To update/refresh the learner with the necessary skills, including breakaway and physical interventions, to improve confidence when managing aggression	See above	See above
Basic life support	To update the learner in basic techniques, maintenance of life support, local policies and procedures	All frontline clinical staff	Annual on wards to supplement 'staying alive'
Intermediate life support	To update the learner in resuscitation techniques, maintain life support, procedures and policies on resuscitation, knowledge and competence in the use of resuscitation equipment, O_2, suction, knowledge of drugs involved in resuscitation	SHOs on commencement, medical emergency responders and core trainers	Annual update

table continues

Table 11.2 *cont'd*

Course	Course details and/or information	For whom	Frequency
Mental Health Act	To provide the necessary training to update the learner with current knowledge of the Mental Health Act (1983)	Frontline clinical staff and social workers	The intention would be that staff received training once every 2 years
Suicide risk assessment and management		All frontline clinical staff	Once every 3 years
First aid	Guidance—at least one first aider per 40 staff but ensure shift coverage	Nominated people	4 days initial programme; 2-day update (every 3 years)
Clinical supervision	To undertake supervision regularly for professional development	All staff	A minimum of 4–6 weeks

A&C, administrative and clerical; AHP, allied health professional; RSU, regional secure unit; SHO, senior house officer; SpR, specialist registrar

for example, in probation or the criminal justice agencies, or from the police or the prison service. What is, of course, important and central to this sort of educational experience would be the bringing together of those with an understanding of the field, an interest in the pursuit of knowledge, and their own background work and experience upon which to draw and to bring to share with others.

One model might be based on a course aimed at experienced practitioners, something that would seem appropriate and desirable, but also which brings with it certain practical difficulties. Simple issues of time and money to put into this form of study over, potentially, a prolonged period of time, for heavily committed and hard-working clinicians, may be a stumbling block. In addition, if one expects to appeal to mature, suitably qualified professionals who are continuing to operate in the relevant field, these are likely to be people for whom the opportunities to study, to read, to assimilate new information and produce written work, may be limited by the requirements of everyday life. One way of helping with this would be to run the proposed course on a part-time basis in a modular, taught form, for instance, on one day or one half-day per week. This would allow students to negotiate their professional work time more readily and, if the day of the week remains consistent throughout the duration of the course, to know when they will need to have their regular time off duty. The use of a modular structure, with the course broken down into discrete units of teaching within a particular subject area, allows for some degree of flexibility and, if there are other similar courses available, for instance, mixing and matching of different elements from parallel programmes. Equally, if the host institution is able to accommodate it, students who are unable, for whatever valid reason, to take a module or complete it, or attend enough of its components to have obtained sufficient teaching to pass, may be able to take the same module at another time or in another year of the course, if there is a rolling programme. The modularised approach also allows for continuous assessment, for instance, by means of student presentations and assignment work linked to the subject in question, which again may be helpful to part-time postgraduate students with substantial work and other commitments.

The subject matter of a multidisciplinary postgraduate course in forensic mental health would never be able to cover everything. The selection of topics offered may depend, to some extent, upon local need and changes in the field in general, but one might argue that there are certain core elements that would have to be included, such as models of service delivery and their historical development, the workings of the criminal justice system and its dealings with the mentally disordered, risk assessment and management, multidisciplinary team working itself and future developments in the field. The content of the course should ideally be adjusted to the needs of those taking it and would also be expected to evolve over time in response to changes in working practice and policy, and alterations in service provision. Again, there may be the need to retain a degree of flexibility about the exact content of each module to keep pace with change and students' requirements.

There is likely to be a research component in a postgraduate degree at the level envisaged here. Many of those coming to such a course may have little or no experience in research previously and consequently appropriate teaching would be necessary. Once more, one of the advantages of a modular course might be that one could then offer qualification at different levels, depending on achievement and individual need and ability. For instance, there may be postgraduate certificates available for completion of a core number of course components, a diploma awarded on successful completion of all core modules and associated assignment work, and a masters-level qualification with successful completion of all taught components, and the production and examination of a dissertation based on a piece of original research.

A course of this nature is likely to be labour intensive and require considerable support, not least in terms of permanent administrative staff and an appropriate academic structure. In addition, it is likely to require input from clinicians working in the field to design and implement it as well as maintain the programme, approach potential speakers and seminar leaders, evaluate and modify teaching and examination methods, and provide academic, personal and pastoral supervision for students. In addition, there is the need to deal with applications, to have sufficient manpower to mark written work, and deal with advertising and recruitment. This sort of undertaking may seem a daunting task but, if multidisciplinary postgraduate education is to have an influence in the field of forensic mental health care, then this may be one way of taking things forward.

PATIENTS AND CARERS IN MULTIDISCIPLINARY EDUCATION

The place of patients, or users, and their carers in relation to a wide variety of areas of health care in general, has gained increasing prominence. As described elsewhere in this book, there has also been a growing emphasis on user, or consumer, involvement in health care research at all levels and specifically, latterly, in the forensic mental health care field. There has been somewhat less emphasis on the involvement of patients and their relatives, family members or carers, in training and teaching activities of health care professionals. It might be argued that this is a particularly important group of people to consider in relation to multi-disciplinary learning in forensic mental health, given the adverse and difficult experiences of many of those who come into contact with such services, but equally, there is a suggestion that has been advanced that users and carers might be considered actually as members of the team at times. The National Service Framework for mental health states clearly that patients ought to be 'involved in planning, providing and evaluating education and training' (Department of Health, 1999). User and carer participation in teaching and learning is likely to be highly enlightening; to lead to improvement of services and be beneficial, if done well, to the individual or individuals concerned themselves. Recently published guidelines have addressed a whole host of reasons why user and carer involvement in training is of value, and also practical issues such as selecting the appropriate person to be involved, what sort of learning experience might be suitable, how to deal with issues such as travel and payment, and also how to avoid or overcome possible difficulties (The National Institute for Mental Health in England (NIMHE) West Midlands Development Centre, 2004). The NIMHE West Midlands Development Centre guidance paper entitled *Involving service users and carers in training* lays out a suggested foundation to 'promote good practice in user and carer mental health act training and development' (NIMHE West Midlands Development Centre, 2004). As well as advantages and disadvantages of this sort of approach, in a wider sense, it addresses specific issues that relate to the potential importance of user and carer involvement in training in the use of mental health legislation, particularly from the point of view of the individual personal experience of the process of assessment for compulsory admission to hospital. The guidance paper does not shy away from difficult areas, such as negative attitudes towards user and carer involvement in training, but offers an optimistic, yet realistic, view of the way forward in involving these most important groups in enhancing professional education.

EVALUATION AND AUDIT

Training in multidisciplinary and interagency working is essential, as will be training in appropriate and timely methods of evaluation and audit. Affara (1997) suggests that learning in a multidisciplinary context will affect the lifelong learning of mental health professionals, where constructive and effective team cohesion in the delivery of effective care should be taught and translated into practice.

Grant (1992) identifies a number of methods of evaluation, which include self-report clinical record audit (independent review of patient's clinical records) and direct observation by an independent professional. Grant's methods are a good starting point for most organisations, however, Thompson et al. (2001) recommend professional development as a mechanism to capture change as the preferred route. The organisation and the professional, through professional development, in attitude, values, as well as a narrower focus on outcomes in a specific area of practice, can be an effective evaluation strategy (Thompson et al., 2001). It is also important that the individual professional is afforded the opportunity to reflect upon learning opportunities in a systematic way by asking themselves a series of pertinent questions.

REFLECTION

- What are the key points I have learned?
- How might these be applied to my practice?
- Are there issues or areas that need further work?
- How well am I using opportunities to share my learning with colleagues?
- Am I getting the most out of my learning?

CONCLUSION

Skeil (1995) asserts that, through more multidisciplinary education and training, there will be greater understanding and communication within teams. If a strategy developed by an organisation for education and training is sound and well grounded, it will ensure that all forensic mental health professionals within it are utilising the best evidence base to inform clinical practice. In continuing to develop a coherent skills and knowledge base, all professional groups may confirm their specific contribution to multidisciplinary working in forensic mental health care. Central to an organisation's success with regard to continuing professional development, is the capacity of a service, to raise the concept and profile of lifelong learning.

It can be said that forensic mental health services retain a substantial number of highly trained professional groups who remain strongly committed to providing the best possible standards of care and treatment to one of the most disadvantaged groups in our society. This collective commitment to providing the best treatment and care to the mentally disordered offender can be enhanced by ensuring that the proper elements of a service-wide education and training programme are in place, and one which has shared ownership.

Finally, forensic mental health services generate and contribute to a substantial body of knowledge related to mental health care, which includes the prevention and treatment of mental disorder, social and criminological responses to offending behaviour, and the development of national standards for the management of mentally disordered offenders.

References

Affara F (1999) Why lifelong learning? International Nursing Review 44: 177–180

Bloom B L and Parad H J (1976) Interdisciplinary training and interdisciplinary functioning: a survey of attitudes and practices in community mental health. American Journal of Orthopsychiatry 46: 669–677

Chaloner C (2000) Characteristics, skills, knowledge and inquiry. In: Chaloner C and Coffey M (eds) Forensic mental health nursing: current approaches. Oxford: Blackwell Science

Department of Health (1997) The new NHS. London: HMSO

Department of Health (1999) Mental health national service framework: modern standards and service models. London: HMSO

Grant R (1992) Obsolescence or lifelong education: choices and challenges. Physiotherapy 78: 167–171

Hope R (1999) Commissioning and provision of training for forensic services in the West Midlands. High Security Psychiatric Services Commissioning Board and NHS Executive West Midlands. Training, Workforce Planning and Education for Working With Mentally Disordered Offenders, West Midlands Regional Seminar. Birmingham: NHS Executive/High Security Commissioning Board

National Health Service Executive (1998) Working together—securing a quality workforce for the NHS. HSC 1998/162. London: Department of Health

NIMHE West Midlands Mental Health Development Centre (2004) Involving service users and carers in training. London: Waterloo Design and Print

Sainsbury Centre for Mental Health (1997) Pulling together, the future roles and training of mental health staff. London: Sainsbury Centre for Mental Health

Skeil D (1995) Individual and staff professional development in a multidisciplinary team: some needs and solutions. Clinical Rehabilitation 9: 28–33

Thomas-Peter B (1999) Treatment integrity and its relationship to training. High Security Psychiatric Services Commissioning Board and NHS Executive West Midlands. Training, Workforce Planning and Education for Working With Mentally Disordered Offenders, West Midlands Regional Seminar. Birmingham: NHS Executive/High Security Commissioning Board

Thompson T, Aiken F and Harvey R (2001) Education and training developments in the context of clinical governance. In: Dale C and Woods P (eds) Forensic mental health issues in practice. London: Balliere Tindall

UKCC and University of Central Lancashire (1999) Nursing in secure environments. London: UKCC

Chapter **12**

Multidisciplinary research

Stuart Wix, Sharon Riordan and Martin Humphreys

INTRODUCTION

Research and development in the National Health Service (NHS) is defined as being activity designed to generate new, potentially universal knowledge, which can be disseminated and subjected to public scrutiny, normally through publication (Department of Health, 1994a). With regard to forensic mental health care, over the years there has been a steady growth in the numbers of papers published, which include those reporting research conducted by a range of different mental health professionals. Despite this, Burrow (1999) suggests that there are relatively few that are the result of truly multidisciplinary collaborations, despite the need for multidisciplinary research being very much on the professional and political agenda over the past decade (Department of Health, 1994b).

It is also important, in the UK context, to consider the need for research in this area in relation to government policy in recent times. In the White paper 'A first class service' (Secretary of State for Health, 1998), the agenda for quality was set, connecting clinical judgement of individual practitioners with clear agreed national standards for health care (Swage, 2000). One of the main components for ensuring high-quality care was said to be: 'The setting of clear standards, including the role of the National Institute for Clinical Excellence and the National Service Frameworks'.

Clinical governance as a framework for improving the quality of clinical care was initially developed for NHS Trusts, and advocated, amongst other principles, that evidence-based practice should be supported and continually applied in everyday practice. According to Clifton and Harvey (2001), evidence-based practice is an approach to decision-making, which draws on four types of information, namely:

- research evidence;
- clinical judgement;
- patient references;
- available resources.

The relatively limited range of multidisciplinary collaborations in research that have been undertaken have resulted in a range of beneficial findings and, therefore, likely clinical outcomes. Research that is more multidisciplinary in nature is, arguably, more likely to be multiperspective, and to address overall service needs and not necessarily individual profession-based deficits. A number of multidisciplinary studies have led to more fundamental and strategic developments in clinical care and service provision (see Brett, 1992; Maden et al., 1993; Riordan et al., 2000; Sumathipala et al., 2003). Multidisciplinary research, in short, reflects how care and treatment is delivered directly to the patient, and by teams, as opposed to some single-discipline studies, which might tend inadvertently to create the impression of working in professional 'silos'. This chapter will attempt to provide a model of how a forensic service might encourage greater multidisciplinary collaboration in research as part of a clear service-related academic and research strategy. An overview of certain aspects of research methodology will be discussed, in particular with reference to multidisciplinary working. Finally, there will be some exploration of the service-user as a potential member of the multidisciplinary research team, and some of the benefits and difficulties that this important issue might raise.

WHERE DO WE START?

Research findings can be classified using the 'hierarchy' of evidence adopted in the National Service Framework (NSF) for Mental Health (Department of Health, 1999) as follows.

- *Type 1*—evidence represents at least one good systematic review, including at least one randomised controlled trial.
- *Type 2*—evidence represents at least one good randomised controlled trial.
- *Type 3*—evidence represents at least one well-designed intervention study without randomisation.
- *Type 4*—evidence represents at least one well-designed observational study.
- *Type 5*—evidence represents expert opinion, including the opinion of service user and carers.

The National Institute for Mental Health in England (NIMHE) commissioned a review of recent literature on adult mental health services, with specific sections focused on forensic mental health. This identified the following areas and issues as being characteristic of the forensic field. (NIMHE, 2003: 3).

- Forensic mental health services are extremely complex, with many different routes in and a wide range of service users.
- Forensic services potentially involve a large number of agencies (such as health care, social care, probation and the prison service).
- By definition, forensic services will be working with people who may display extremely challenging behaviours and who may have been found to be too difficult to work with within other settings prior to their referral to forensic care.

The review also highlighted three main issues that were considered to be in need of further investigation (NIMHE, 2003: 4):

- the level of unmet mental health needs in prison;
- the level of inappropriate placements in secure services;
- the need for greater partnership working.

UNMET MENTAL HEALTH NEEDS IN PRISON

It has been established now for some considerable time that there are a large number of people with unmet mental health needs in prison, both on remand and as sentenced prisoners, despite the emphasis placed on diverting people with mental health problems away from the criminal justice system where possible and practicable. NIMHE suggested that there is growing evidence in the literature, which raises serious questions about the role that prisons may be being asked to play in caring for people with mental health problems, and the extent to which prisons and prison staff are equipped, or not, to fulfil this role.

THE LEVEL OF INAPPROPRIATE PLACEMENTS IN SECURE SETTINGS

NIHME went on to express concern that the increasingly inappropriate use of existing bed capacity in secure services as a whole may be as a consequence of the high levels of unmet health needs in prison. A number of studies have highlighted the substantial delays in admitting patients to low-secure services from medium security, or from prison to medium or high security, owing to a lack of alternative services for long-stay patients who were considered inappropriate for placement in general psychiatric rehabilitation units. Therefore, difficulties encountered with discharging patients to lower levels of security can also make it harder to admit patients who require care in a more secure environment.

THE NEED FOR GREATER PARTNERSHIP WORKING

NIMHE argued that, despite the considerable barriers to working in partnership that the literature suggests, there is a need for a clear pathway from the point of entry into a forensic service, through to the point of discharge, incorporating community and mainstream mental health care providers. In short, the provision of effective mental health services requires a wide range of agencies to work closely together, and the review suggested that research in the field in future should embrace this approach too. Although individual services have unique issues to examine and perhaps evaluate, it is clear that there are wider national and 'systems' research-related issues that ought to be pursued.

However, it is of vital importance that the research agenda is tackled in a collaborative, systematic and multidisciplinary manner. This can be achieved through the mechanism of a multiprofessional academic and research forum or committee, with clearly defined and agreed terms of reference. These might include for instance:

- a regular monthly meeting;
- encouragement of research within the service by making it both more accessible to a wider range of professions, and offering support and advice during all stages of the research process;
- service development of a research strategy and agenda aligned with local, regional and national priorities;
- peer review of research proposals;
- regular reviews of the impact of research on clinical practice and service delivery;
- pooling of diverse multidisciplinary research expertise, and appropriate allocation of research resources and sources of funding.

A multidisciplinary academic and research committee, if run equitably and consistently over time, can have a positive effect upon the quality of projects undertaken, their number, the focus of research activity within a given service and the culture of the service itself. Well-established committees may be able to assist in tackling inequalities that exist amongst professions who have varying abilities and inclination to conduct research, and also experience, expertise and a research 'culture'.

The nursing profession, for example, is one discipline where there might be said to be a lack of confidence and, to some extent, the required academic rigour to allow large numbers of its members to embark on research projects successfully. This is borne out by a recent study of nursing in secure environments (UKCC and University of Central Lancashire, 1999), which found that, despite forensic nurses claiming that an evidence base was used to inform their practice, the evidence cited and employed tended to be anecdotal and experiential rather than research related. The lack of competent experienced researchers amongst the nursing profession is a serious issue. Change is only likely to come about as a result of provision of accessible professional education to suit local purposes, as well as other experience in clinical audit, research and development activities and support systems, and in addition, investment in training, which is preferably multidisciplinary. The literature also suggests that nursing as a profession does not yet have a 'culture' of research interest or research utilisation, and that the environment of more closed institutions does not necessarily promote changes in practice to take on board research evidence (United Kingdom Central Council for Nursing, Midwifery and Health Visiting (UKCC) and University of Central Lancashire, 1999), something which is likely to have an obvious impact in forensic settings.

A multidisciplinary academic and research committee can, therefore, potentially also develop strategies to support and train those disciplines, including nursing, which have not, historically, had extensive experience in research, through incremental exposure to research activity, through involvement in short projects with a straightforward research design, to participation in more complex and prolonged studies, which require a collaborative team approach.

QUANTITY AND QUALITY IN MULTIDISCIPLINARY RESEARCH IN FORENSIC MENTAL HEALTH CARE

The *Research governance framework for England* (1st edn, Autumn 2001; Department of Health, 2001) confirms that research is essential to the successful promotion of health and well-being. During the last century, major advances have depended on research and, ever increasingly, professionals from all disciplines, service users, carers and the general public are progressively looking to research for additional improvements in the development and delivery of health and social care services.

The subsequent *Research governance framework for health and social care* (2nd edn, Autumn 2003; Department of Health, 2003) set standards to help improve research quality whilst simultaneously safeguarding the public by aiming to create a research environment of greater integrity through the promotion of high standards, and stringent monitoring and assessment procedures. Overall, the implementation of research governance is intended to ensure that the quality of research undertaken in health and social care is improved by enhancing the ethical and scientific quality, endorsing good practice, lessening the likelihood of adverse incidents and, where problems occur, making certain that lessons are learned, culminating in the elimination of poor performance and misconduct (Department of Health, 2003: 2). Importantly, in the interest of multidisciplinary collaboration, the framework remains grounded on principles that may be applied to an extensive range of research designs and contexts.

Health and social care services are unique in that staff from both disciplines consistently work across professional and organisational margins, something which is particularly evident in the multidisciplinary team within forensic services. Consequently, over time, a great deal of expertise and good practice is accumulated. The problem that arises in multidisciplinary partnerships is that, although all disciplines have the best interests of service users and their carers at their core; in reality the different disciplines have different priorities, cultures and indeed language (Moullin, 2002). This can have particular consequences for the development of multidisciplinary research in forensic mental health care as a whole. Nevertheless, undertaking collaborative research in forensic services where individuals work across organisational boundaries can have research benefits for all those involved, as it lessens the overlap between services and the communication difficulties often associated with distinctly separate departments.

One of the main considerations for multidisciplinary researchers is which research method to choose. Traditionally, research in health has been the domain of the medical profession and the debate about the superiority of quantitative and qualitative research methods has stemmed from the desire to underpin progress in the natural sciences that is 'the scientific method'. However, recently, health services have become more accepting of qualitative approaches and methods that explicitly link social issues and professional practice.

Quantitative and qualitative research methods are often presented as polarised epistemological viewpoints presenting different ways of knowing the social world. Quantitative research methods derive from the positivist approach of the 16th and 17th century that emphasised precise measurement, causality generalisation and replication. The philosophy that underpins positivism, therefore, is the assumption that what cannot be observed and numerically measured is not open to scientific investigation (Coolican, 1996). Social research taking a positivist approach has centred on the behaviour of groups of people, and has taken no account of individual experiences, values and attitudes. In response to the rigid interpretation of scientific research, Harré (1981) concluded that positivism has led to a vast amount of superficial, irrelevant data and theory. The more traditional research paradigm (Kuhn, 1962) has characteristics that are often objected to by those in search of a more qualitative approach to human investigation. It suggests that conventional research isolates people, and parts of people from the surrounding context with subjects thought of as indistinguishable units able to be manipulated in and out of the research condition. It is expected that researchers are to remain distant from their subjects and their personal attitudes. The assumed objectivity within the traditional paradigm has been described as imaginary as the research environment is a social situation where people interact. The experimental context does not allow the subjects freedom to react in a natural way and express suitable social behaviour, yet the data generated are seen as realistic and generalisable. This situation has resulted in an oversimplistic mechanistic model of human behaviour.

In the health field—an area with a strong tradition of biomedical research using conventional, quantitative and very often experimental methods—qualitative research is regularly criticised on the grounds of the lack of scientific rigour and credibility. The most commonly voiced criticism is that qualitative research is simply a collection of anecdotal and personal impressions subject to researcher bias (Mays and Pope, 1995). It has also been suggested that qualitative research lacks reproducibility because it is so individual to the researcher that there can be no guarantee that a different investigator would not come to completely different conclusions. Stanley and Wise (1983: 179) asserted 'Research is the process which occurs through the medium of a person—the researcher is always and inevitably present in the research'. Efforts have been made to address this criticism. One possible solution is to read back the narrative to the research participant to ensure the fairness and integrity of the researcher, and to check communicative validity (Gaskell and Beauer, 1992). Another way of tackling the problem is to make the data available to the reader on computer disc (Mays and Pope, 1995).

Doctors have historically placed a premium on numerical data, which some have suggested, in reality, might be criticised as ambiguous, reductionist and to a great extent irrelevant to the real issues. The mounting recognition of the role of qualitative research methods in the biomedical sciences has occurred because of the limitations inherent in the use of quantitative research methods that have resulted, in some cases, in incorrect answers to significant questions in the areas of clinical care and service delivery (Black, 1994). Although the qualitative methods found more commonly in the social sciences may appear unfamiliar alongside the quantitative methods more traditionally used in clinical and biomedical research, they should be viewed as a vital component of health and social care research (Mays and Pope, 1995).

There can be no doubt that the range of qualitative research methods including in-depth interviews, ethnography and observation are important to those researchers who seek a deeper truth (Greenhalgh and Taylor, 1997). Qualitative methods are primarily useful when there is a desire to appreciate the meanings and interpretation of different facets of health and social care by drawing on the experiences of those being studied. Qualitative methods are particularly useful to illuminate how individuals perceive social systems and how those social systems function in a natural context (Ziebland and Wright, 1997; Riordan et al., 2003, 2004). It might be argued that this is particularly important in a multidisciplinary setting and way of working.

Qualitative research methods are being used much more extensively now in, for example, nursing research and evaluation (Wright, 1998; Lawler et al., 1999) and, more recently, there have been strenuous efforts made by some to advocate the value of qualitative research methods to a diverse audience in health and social services research (Pope and Mays, 1995). Qualitative research methods have been utilised in social and educational research and medical sociology for a considerable time. In 1994, Fitzpatrick and Boulton raised awareness of the stimulating range of qualitative methods capable of providing a basic understanding of the processes and outcomes of health care.

Nonetheless, the concerns about qualitative research methods are still evident and, to some extent, have led to different ways of combining both methods of data collection without compromising their diverse derivations (Grbich, 1999). Generally, the aim is to seek an amalgamation of the data that are said to enhance research validity and establish a more complete picture of an experience by combining diverse perspectives (Grbich, 1999).

There have, therefore, been a number of attempts to combine quantitative and qualitative research methods. Pradilla's (1992) research was based on a parallel methods approach where the results of two similar but separately located studies were triangulated. Triangulation involves overlapping results at several points to improve reliability. The quantitative study utilised a researcher-developed, piloted, factor-analysed questionnaire to investigate students' perceptions of their academic tutors. Factor analysis is an approach that makes sense of a great number of correlations between variables. There is a similarity between this and multiple logistic regression analysis, but it differs in that the variables under examination all have equal status and no individual variable is designated as the dependent variable. Factor analysis begins with a matrix of correlations (Robson, 2002). Matrices of this type are difficult to interpret, particularly when they contain large quantities of variables. Factor analysis aims to replace a large and unmanageable set of variables with a small and straightforwardly understood number of factors (Robson, 2002). A factor-analysed questionnaire, therefore, is a product of a series of factors in numerical order. The results derived from the quantitative study included academic and socioemotional skills and level of knowledge as important factors influencing student perceptions of their tutors. The qualitative part of the study used interviews that were analysed through a process of concept modelling to identify types of tutors, what they do, their style of delivery, and the relationship between tutor and student. Concept modelling involves connecting an assortment of concepts under one theme in order to emphasise a specific perspective (Grbich, 1999). Pradilla's study pointed to the consistency of the results and, therefore, to the potential of convergent triangulation.

Other studies have attempted to gain a wider view through the triangulation of two sets of data, both quantitative and qualitative, using the same research question from the same respondents in a single study. Prein (1992) investigated associations between women's professional career decisions and their family biographies. The qualitative interviews found that family factors had the foremost impact on decision-making. The quantitative data derived from cluster analysis and suggested that a specific profession, not family factors, was the primary causal component in the women's decision-making. Therefore, in this example, the researchers viewed the two sets of data as wholly contradictory.

Mason's (1994) research used two data sets, one quantitative and one qualitative, to explore the same topic. A large-scale survey of 978 respondents was undertaken to investigate what people thought they should do for their relatives in order to create an extensive picture. This was followed by semistructured face-to-face interviews to elicit the differing aspects of meaning on the topic. In this particular research, the purpose of two data sets was not to attempt triangulation but to access information on various levels of meaning.

It could be argued that combining quantitative and qualitative research methods allows the researcher to examine both hard and soft data and, in the context of multidisciplinary health and social care teams, allows expression of the different interests and cultures within disciplines. Diverse investigative positions are associated with different types of knowledge and it is individuals who create hierarchies in research by conferring legitimacy to one type of knowledge over another (Stevenson and Cooper, 1997). By embracing the perspective of research that encompasses a reflective and open-minded approach, to enable the suitable selection of appropriate research methods for the phenomena under investigation and the analysis of the findings, this may become one of the key principles for high-quality multidisciplinary research in forensic services.

Qualitative methods are being used more regularly to investigate reasonably complex issues for considerate and meticulous analysis. One of the main strengths of the qualitative approach in multidisciplinary health and social care research is that some of the insights the research reveals can often '. . . expose unanticipated layers of complexity rather than provide final answers' (Ziebland and Wright, 1997: 124).

Perhaps the most constructive indicator of the credibility of research findings is when, practitioners, service users, carers and the public can examine the findings and consider them relevant in terms of their experiences. Fundamentally though, research undertaken in health and social care, in whatever context, and by whichever research methods, should strive to meet stringent standards set by research governance and always have the interests of the research subjects, or participants, as the prime consideration. It must be clearly illustrated that all those involved in research have taken the exhaustive steps necessary to protect the rights, dignity, safety and overall well-being of all those involved.

USER INVOLVEMENT IN FORENSIC MENTAL HEALTH RESEARCH

As previously described, the service user, or patient, is always central to the work of the multidisciplinary team and may even be considered as part of it. One way in which this has been brought out as being particularly important in recent times is in relation to the involvement of users, consumers, patrons or patients in health care research in general and, more specifically, in the field of forensic mental health.

Some areas of health care have involved carers and patients very actively in seeking and advising on views in relation to the provision of services and, as a logical extension of that, in research at various different levels. This has tended, in the past, to have involved those groups or individuals who were perhaps most articulate and able to express views clearly, and challenge the medical and allied establishment more readily. Nevertheless, there has been a clear recognition that all user or consumer groups and individuals should be entitled to involvement in health care research programmes and, as a result, the Standing Advisory Group on Consumer Involvement in the NHS Research and Development Programme was established and commenced work in 1996 (NHS Research and Development Programme, 1997). Since that time, the Consumers in NHS Research Support Unit has been established and a Standing Group on Consumers in NHS Research produces regular reports. These have included discussion and descriptions of the reasons why it might be important to involve consumers in research, for instance, in terms of identifying priorities, setting the research agenda and defining clear objectives for project work. In addition, the Standing Group has outlined various research projects involving consumers at the various different levels of possible involvement, from consultation to active participation, and sought to assist in suggesting ways to overcome possible difficulties in involving patients in research partnerships (NHS Executive, 1999; Department of Health, 2000).

Various sources have identified the need for change in terms of patient involvement in research from experimental 'subjects' to co-workers, investigators and colleagues (Goodare and Lockwood, 1999; Trivedi and Wykes, 2002). This suggests a move away from the notion that patients or service users are simply passive recipients to be tested or investigated, towards a model of active consultation to identify matters of importance to consumers, to identify desired outcomes, to improve and to allow wider and more meaningful dissemination of findings through detailed collaboration and, ultimately, user control over research design, methods, analysis, publication and presentation. There has already been work undertaken to determine to what extent patients are involved in this process, within the United Kingdom at least (Hanley et al., 2001), and equally to address the issue specifically of how mental health service users perceive what might be the most important areas to be investigated (Thornicroft et al., 2002). Work involving the active participation of mental health service consumers in research and how this might be of benefit has also been reported in North America (Rogers et al., 1997).

In the particular area of consumer involvement in research and development in the field of mental health, and more specifically that of forensic mental health, there are inevitably hurdles to be overcome, but also potential benefits as already outlined. There may be issues around confidentiality, whether patients are representative of a particular group as a whole, or whether those suffering from the more severe forms of mental disorder and mental illness are able, as a result of their symptoms and need for treatment, to collaborate and be involved effectively. In addition, as in other fields, there might be particular patients or groups of patients who have specific reasons for wishing to challenge the traditional methods of research and investigation; very often this will be a good thing, but might create its own difficulties. There is, in this more general context, also the matter of overcoming possibly entrenched attitudes among health care professionals in relation to sharing of expertise and resources as well as relinquishing, at least to some extent, control over research and its use (Hanley et al., 2001).

In the field of mental health care and, in particular, with patients involved with forensic services and in secure settings, or subject to compulsory detention, there may be major issues to be considered in relation to insight and working with clinician researchers in circumstances where involuntary measures or interventions might predominate (Adshead and Brown, 2003). Despite this, in the United Kingdom, the National Health Service Programme on Forensic Mental Health Research and Development has published an expert paper entitled *User involvement in forensic mental health research and development*, clearly setting out an agenda with, at its centre, the aim of involving patients or consumers and their carers in research and development in the field (Faulkner and Morris, 2003). This is an important and informative document that seeks to address the reasons why user involvement in forensic mental health care research might be of benefit, but does not shy away from raising the potential difficulties that might hamper or even in some circumstances prevent this, including the attitudes of professionals in the field and also potential problems in engaging in research in involving patients in a secure environment, for instance, without compromising safety or confidentiality. The authors discuss how involving service users in forensic mental health research might improve quality and validity of findings and the current evidence and its subsequent use, how patients might be more able, from a background of personal experience, to define appropriate research questions, and how this might benefit the individual patient, researcher and the institution as a whole, as a result of increasing mutual respect and levels of involvement. They also discuss the potential pitfalls, not least issues around gaining access to a relatively small and potentially physically confined group of patients who may already have been subject to research, difficulties in overcoming staff attitudes, concerns again over security and the management of risk and the issues about misunderstandings and perceived imposition of further requirements on already, in some cases, resistant and potentially oppositional, ill individuals. Faulkner and Morris (2003) give a number of examples of areas where user involvement in mental health research is already under way and describe some of the issues already addressed. They go some way to pointing to future directions for this type of work.

Given the nature of the field, it would seem to make sense that those patients involved with forensic services, who may be subject to particularly restrictive measures and requirements, should be encouraged and actively assisted in becoming involved in health care research, should they wish to do so. Nevertheless, attempts to pursue this may prove difficult at first for a variety of reasons. This will hopefully not, however, prevent the continued development of programmes intended to involve service users at all levels and, in particular, in collaboration with already experienced investigators, which, it might be argued, is likely to improve future efforts to continue this sort of work and break down barriers.

CONCLUSION

This chapter has described how forensic mental health services might engage in opportunities to conduct research in a more collaborative way. There is a relative dearth of published multidisciplinary research in relation to forensic mental health care, yet there is a growing body of evidence that highlights the value of conducting studies that are collaborative in nature. Clinical practice enhancement and the improvement of health outcomes for service users in forensic settings are, therefore, imperative for the continued benefit of individual patients, clinicians and researchers, and for the progression of services nationally.

References

Adshead G and Brown C (2003) Ethical issues in forensic mental health research. London: Jessica Kingsley

Black N (1994) Why we need qualitative research. Journal of Epidemiology and Community Health 48: 425–426

Brett T (1992) Treatment in secure hospitals. Criminal Behaviour and Mental Health 2: 152–158

Burrow S (1999) The forensic multidisciplinary team. In: Tarbuck P, Topping Morris B and Burnard P (eds) Forensic mental health nursing, strategy and implication. London: Whurr Publishers

Clifton M and Harvey R (2001) Evidence-based practice and clinical monitoring. In: Dale C, Thompson T and Woods P (eds) Forensic mental health issues in practice. London: Balliere Tindall

Coolican H (1996) Introduction to research methods and statistics in psychology, 2nd edn. London: Hodder and Stoughton

Department of Health (1994a) Supporting research and development in the NHS (The Culyer Report). London: HMSO

Department of Health (1994b) Working in partnership. London: HMSO

Department of Health (1999) National service framework for mental health: modern standards and service models. London: HMSO

Department of Health (2000) Consumers in NHS Research, 3rd annual report. Working partnerships. London: HMSO

Department of Health (2001) Research governance framework for England, Autumn. London: HMSO

Department of Health (2003) Research governance framework for health and social care, 2nd edn, Autumn. London: HMSO

Faulkner A and Morris B (2003) User involvement in forensic mental health research and development. Liverpool: NHS National Programme on Forensic Mental Health Research and Development

Fitzpatrick R and Boulton M (1994) Qualitative methods for assessing health care. Quality in Health Care 3: 107–113

Gaskell G and Beauer M W (1992) Towards public accountability: beyond sampling, reliability and validity. In: Beauer M W and Gaskell G (eds) Qualitative research with text, image and sound: a practical handbook. London: Sage Publications

Goodare H and Lockwood S (1999) Involving patients in clinical research. British Medical Journal 319: 724–725

Grbich C (1999) Qualitative research in health: an introduction. London: Sage Publications

Greenhalgh T and Taylor R (1997) How to read a paper: papers that go beyond numbers (qualitative research). British Medical Journal 315: 740–743

Hanley B, Truesdale A, King A, Elbourne D and Chalmers I (2001) Involving consumers in designing, constructing, and interpreting randomised controlled trials: questionnaire survey. British Medical Journal 322: 519–523

Harré R (1981) The positivist-empiricist approach and its alternative. In: Reason R and Rowan J (eds) Human inquiry: a sourcebook of new paradigm research. Chichester: Wiley

Kuhn T (1962) The structure of scientific revolutions. Chicago: University of Chicago Press

Lawler J, Dowswell G, Hearn J, Forster A and Young J (1999) Recovering from stroke: a qualitative investigation of the role of goal setting in late stroke recovery. Journal of Advanced Nursing 30: 401–409

Maden A, Curle C, Meux C, Burrow S and Gunn J (1993) Treatment and security needs of special hospitals patients. London: Whurr Publishers

Mason J (1994) Linking qualitative and quantitative data. In: Bryman A and Burgess R G (eds) Analyzing qualitative data. London: Routledge

Mays N and Pope C (1995) Qualitative research: rigour and qualitative research. British Medical Journal 311: 109–112

Moullin M (2002) Delivering excellence in health and social care. Buckingham: Open University Press

NHS Executive (1999) The second report of the Standing Group on Consumers in the NHS Research. Involvement works. London: NHS Executive

NHS Research and Development Programme (1997) Report of the Standing Advisory Group on Consumer Involvement in the NHS Research and Development Programme. Health research: what's in it for consumers? London: NHS Research and Development Programme

NIMHE (2003) Cases for change: a review of the foundations of mental health policy and practice 1997–2002. London: Department of Health

Pope C and Mays N (1995) Qualitative research: reaching parts other methods cannot reach: an introduction to qualitative methods in health and social services research. British Medical Journal 311: 42–45

Pradilla R (1992) Qualitative and quantitative models of social situations: the case for triangulation of paradigms. Cited in Grbich (1999)

Prien G (1992) Traps of triangulation: what can be done by combining quantitative and qualitative research methods? Cited in Grbich (1999)

Riordan S, Wix S, Kenney-Herbert J and Humphreys M (2000) Diversion at the point of arrest: a description of mentally disordered individuals early contact with the police in Birmingham. Journal of Forensic Psychiatry 3: 683–690

Riordan S, Smith H and Humphreys M (2002) Alternative perceptions of statutory community aftercare: patient and responsible medical officer views. Journal of Mental Health Law No 7: 119–129

Riordan S, Donaldson S and Humphreys M (2004) The imposition of restricted hospital orders: potential effects of ethnic origin. International Journal of Law and Psychiatry 27: 171–177

Robson C (2002) Real world research. Oxford: Blackwell

Rogers E S, Chamberlin J, Ellison M L and Crean B (1997) A consumer scale to measure empowerment among users of mental health services. Psychiatric Services 48: 1042–1047

Secretary of State for Health (1998) A first class service, quality in the new NHS. London: NHS Executive

Stanley L and Wise S (1983) Breaking out: feminist consciousness and feminist research. London: Routledge and Kegan Paul

Stevenson C and Cooper N (1997) Qualitative and quantitative research. The Psychologist 10: 220–229

Sumathipala A, Siribaddana S, Sumaraweera S and Dayaratne D (2003) Capacity building through multi-disciplinary research. British Journal of Psychiatry 183: 457–458

Swage T (2000) Clinical governance in healthcare practice. Oxford: Butterworth Heinemann

Thornicroft G, Rose D, Huxley P, Dale G and Wykes T (2002) What are the research priorities of mental health service users? Journal of Mental Health 11: 1–5

Trivedi P and Wykes T (2002) From passive subjects to equal partners. British Journal of Psychiatry 181: 468–472

UKCC and University of Central Lancashire (1999) Nursing in secure environments. London: UKCC

Wright S (1998) Changing nursing practice. London: Arnold

Ziebland S and Wright L (1997) Qualitative research methods. In: Jenkinson C (ed.) Assessment and evaluation of health and social care: a methods text. Buckingham: Open University Press

Conclusions and the way ahead

Stuart Wix and Martin Humphreys

This book has been about multidisciplinary working in forensic mental health care. The use of the term forensic health care itself is an indication that the field involves more than a single discipline and that the provision of services is now more inclusive and wider reaching. We have aimed to give an historical overview of the background to the development of this way of working, to define what teamwork is, to show how that teamwork might translate into effective, focused clinical practice, to touch on potential team membership, and the types of team-building activities that can be engaged in to develop and enhance team functioning. We have also described some areas related to research and development, as well as teaching and other educational activities.

Team working in health care, in general, is the modern-day gold standard. Multidisciplinary and multiagency working is the accepted norm in forensic mental health care and, therefore, well developed both in principle and practice. Nevertheless, this is still a developing area of work. Despite the ideal, there is considerable progress to be made and little room for complacency. It is commonplace to find a whole variety of barriers, or potential barriers, to the certainty of fully integrated multiprofessional collaborative practice. In the more distant past, the 'team' has been seen very much as a small core of powerful specialist clinicians. However, over the years, there has been an incremental growth in the professional composition of teams, and increasing involvement with, for example, non-health care agencies. More recently, the impetus has been towards even greater inclusiveness, in partnership with voluntary organisations and their representatives, service users, consumers and carers.

Effective multidisciplinary working has been described in the following way: 'The structure and functioning of teams should depend primarily upon the identified needs of the individual, group or population receiving the service, not upon tradition, charisma or dogma' (British Psychological Society, 1986).

According to Øvretveit (1986), the organisation of team activities and functioning is often viewed by team members and senior management as a peripheral issue or as 'something that will sort itself out'. One of the most important reasons behind team working in health care is to ensure that the skills of different professionals can be easily and swiftly combined to meet the specific needs of a particular individual or client group. This form of organisation is, therefore, crucial for effective teamwork and for providing a high-quality and effective service for patients (Øvretveit, 1986). Team organisation is a complex issue and one that is often neglected. This can result in clinicians sometimes struggling with major difficulties, which might have been resolved had those involved agreed and mapped out basic elements of effective functioning. If this aspect of multidisciplinary working is ignored or goes unrecognised, the consequences are likely to be widespread and enduring. This is particularly relevant in a field where good-quality clinical risk assessment and management are crucial, and where the issues of safety for all those concerned are so vital, and where any adverse incidents will have such profound costs. Effective communication, fostered by close professional collaboration, can only really come out of open, honest and equitable working relationships, within the context of the multidisciplinary clinical team.

We would argue that it is crucial for multidisciplinary team members to be able to set aside dedicated time to establish the appropriate service specification, and agree structure and process for its delivery. Equally there should be clear arrangements in place for overall and individual workload management, supervision and personal development. Consideration must be given to issues such as training, style of leadership, group dynamics and specific operational systems for service evaluation and data recording. Defining structures, boundaries, and team and service objectives are particularly important in view of the emotionally demanding nature of working in a secure setting. All of this requires the commitment of senior management, at all levels, to team working in order to foster the development of new types of service provision and facilitate professional practice that is evidence based. Of course, team members themselves must also be willing to embrace the principles of true, multidisciplinary, multiprofessional practice fully. Øvretveit (1986) asserts that clear structure and objectives are necessary to provide a context within which cooperation and creativity can flourish, where professional staff are more able to concentrate their energies on relieving suffering, and on improving the quality of life of patients and their carers.

There are a number of assumptions associated with the multidisciplinary team model:

- the therapeutic effect of teamwork is greater than the sum of its parts;
- each individual has a particular area of competence;
- team members will share a similar degree of autonomy.

There are, however, as already described in this book, some potential problems associated with this concept. The contributions of individual team members, in terms of professional expertise and personal style may be compromised or lost if the overall emphasis is on democratic majority-based decision-making. Lack of a consensus view about respective roles, professional working practices, and individual and collective areas of responsibility, with the potential for confusion of function, may hinder the overall performance of the team. Other difficulties may arise from differences in professional training, philosophy and levels of experience, and the extent of each member's involvement with their own professional group outside of the team. Ill-feeling between team members, where perhaps a manager is not closely involved, frank disagreement on a clinical issue or where team members are unable to cooperate, will undermine effective collaborative effort.

Although there are these and other potential pitfalls related to team working, they are not necessarily insurmountable. The examples given elsewhere here of exercises to help resolve friction within teams may help to overcome some of the tensions and unhelpful dynamics that do occur from time to time. The successful operation of a multidisciplinary team might be said to depend upon creating a suitable forum where divergent or even diametrically opposed views can safely be represented in discussion, and also be heard by others, and successfully resolved into a broad-based coherent plan of action. Consensus within a team may not always be possible. The outcome may be dependent upon a number of variables. These may include issues around professional responsibility and expertise. Each team member's professional practice should be open to reasonable rational challenge, with access to a mechanism whereby an alternative opinion may be sought (Dale et al., 2001).

There are a number of new developments on the horizon facing forensic mental health care services. One clearly in the public domain is the improvement of services for people with a severe personality disorder, particularly in cases where individuals with this diagnosis are deemed to present a risk to others. This group is likely to present a considerable challenge to good multidisciplinary team working, where clinical effectiveness may be compromised, if the therapeutic approach is inconsistent and team structures are weak. Clinical teams will need to develop further their ability to work in a flexible, but coherent and fully integrated manner.

Another development in services that needs to be addressed urgently relates to changes in the delivery of prison health care, particularly for those suffering from mental illness and other forms of mental disorder. This is now delivered through a formal partnership between the NHS and the Prison Service, but is beset with the inherent difficulties associated with ingrained institutionalised practices. As already outlined in this book, multidisciplinary working in the penal system is a complex and developing sphere of practice, and one that is fraught with problems as services strive to deliver standards of health care comparable to those available in the wider community. The principle of the multidisciplinary approach in areas more traditionally seen as the preserve of individual professional groups, such as training and research, should be firmly grasped. This is something that is likely to require considerable effort and practical application if it is to prove successful in enhancing practice and patient care. The inclusion of service users and carers in all aspects of forensic mental health care service delivery and practice presents a particularly important but also potentially testing area of work. Forensic mental health care services continue to grow apace, which in itself may present a significant barrier to effective multidisciplinary team functioning. In reality, there are more challenges facing those working in the field now than ever before.

References

British Psychological Society (1986) Responsibility issues in clinical psychology and multi-disciplinary teamwork. A report by the Division of Clinical Psychology. London: British Psychological Society

Dale C, Thompson T and Woods P (2001) Forensic mental health issues in practice. London: Balliere Tindall

Øvetveit J (1986) Organisation of multi-disciplinary community teams: a Health Services Centre working paper. London: Brunel Institute of Organisational and Social Studies

Index